Endorsements

The Maker's Diet is a refreshing change in a world full of fad diet books that push unsubstantiated programs, each conflicting with the other. Jordan Rubin derives his health program from the most ancient of public health texts—the Bible. Many of his recommendations have been gleaned from epidemiological studies on some of the world's healthiest people and thus are based on history and proven by modern science. I have taught these principles to patients and students for decades, as well as applying them in my own life. *The Maker's Diet* can serve as an important guide to those seeking to restore or preserve their health.

—Paul A. Goldberg, M.P.H, D.C, D.A.C.B.N, director of The Goldberg Clinic for Chronic Disease Reversal

As a race, man becomes progressively more ill despite the steady growth of the healthcare profession to a multibillion-dollar-per-year industry. And we keep searching for new things to instill health. What about going back to a time when man did truly live healthy, with recorded longevity way beyond that of modern times, and applying those tenets? This, through astounding personal experience and a wealth of knowledge, is exactly what Jordan Rubin has done and explicitly shares with you in *The Maker's Diet*, a must-read for anyone desiring to live a healthy life.

—Marty Goldstein, D.V.M., founder of the Smith Ridge Veterinary Center and author of *The Nature of Animal Healing*

Jordan's faith-based journey from near death to vital health bears witness to the power of pure food prepared in simple, traditional ways that reveal the true spirit of culinary and cooking experiences. Chefs everywhere, heal thyself with *The Maker's Diet*!

—Charles H. Halliday, former president of the Florida Culinary Institute

The Maker's Diet is the answer to the many questions surrounding weight loss and health. This ancient but relevant formula for healthy living and nutritional science is just what Jordan Rubin has recommended for thousands of patients with unbelievable results. Diets come and go, but this cutting-edge program is a must for anyone who is serious about optimal weight management with a practical approach to overall health.

—Terry Lyles, Ph.D., performance psychologist and author of
The Secret to Navigating Life's Storms

Jordan Rubin is a true teacher who brings to us health and nutrition wisdom uncovered from the ages. Read his books and put his wisdom into action for your own life, and you will be healthier.

—David Steinman, publisher of Healthy Living magazine and author of
Diet for a Poisoned Planet and *The Safe Shopper's Bible*

As a coach and trainer, I realize the importance of proper nutrition in the quest for optimum performance. Jordan Rubin's commonsense yet science-based approach to health and nutrition is clearly illustrated in *The Maker's Diet*. However, I believe the best illustration of the power of the Maker's Diet is his own triumph over a life-threatening illness. The Institute of Human Performance is proud to recommend *The Maker's Diet* to everyone from professional athletes to rehab patients.

—Juan Carlos Santana, M.Ed, CSCS, founder of the Institute of Human
Performance and author of *Functional Training,*
Breaking the Bonds of Traditionalism

Jordan is a man of great integrity with a real passion to help people. Not only is Jordan's story remarkable, but also his health program is absolutely outstanding and has been proven with the test of time. *The Maker's Diet* has helped transform my life as well as the lives of my family and many in our congregation.

—Thomas D. Mullins, pastor and founder of Palm Beach Gardens Christ
Fellowship in Palm Beach Gardens, Florida

Quite simply put, *The Maker's Diet* has transformed my family's health. The results of being on this journey with Jordan Rubin have been nothing short of amazing. If your desire is to be healthy and have optimum power in achieving a full and successful life, the Maker's Diet is for you!

—Michael Neale, artist and songwriter of "Your Great Name"

In *The Maker's Diet*, Jordan Rubin brilliantly combines biblical wisdom, scientific knowledge, practical solutions, and his own personal life experience to guide us on a path that leads to good health. This book is fascinating and easy to read. It is a must-read for anyone who desires to live longer and healthier.

—Rabbi Dr. Charles Ian Kluge, former president of the Messianic Jewish Alliance of America

In a world of over-processed, bioengineered, "convenience" foods and fad diets fraught with myths and hype, the modern American diet has proven to be headed down the wrong path. Jordan Rubin's 40-day health experience brilliantly leads us back to the original diet intended for us by our Creator. I will get this timeless and powerfully life-changing book into the hands of everyone I know.

—Ginger Lea Southall, D.C., chiropractic physician, author, and medical TV correspondent

I want to know as much as possible to be healthier and perform optimally as a person and as a professional. With all of the diets on the market, all of the opinions, it gets really confusing. Jordan Rubin's diet makes sense! His book contains practical information on diet, exercise, and all aspects of health. *The Maker's Diet* is very user friendly and written by someone who practices what he preaches.

—Scott Sharp, former Indy Car driver

the
MAKER'S
DIET

UPDATED & EXPANDED

DESTINY IMAGE BOOKS BY JORDAN RUBIN

Essential Fasting
with Josh Axe

The Beginner's Guide to Essential Oils

Essential Oils
with Josh Axe and Ty Bollinger

Patient Heal Thyself

Planet Heal Thyself

Maker's Diet Meals

The Joseph Blessing
with Pete Sulack

Re-size America

The Maker's Diet Revolution

the MAKER'S DIET

UPDATED & EXPANDED

the **40-DAY** *health experience that will change your life forever*

JORDAN RUBIN

DESTINY IMAGE® PUBLISHERS, INC.

P.O. Box 310, Shippensburg, PA 17257-0310

"Promoting Inspired Lives."

This book and all other Destiny Image and Destiny Image Fiction books are available at Christian bookstores and distributors worldwide.

Cover design by Koechel Peterson & Associates

Interior design by Terry Clifton

For more information on foreign distributors, call 717-532-3040.

Reach us on the Internet: www.destinyimage.com.

ISBN 13 TP: 978-0-7684-5626-4

ISBN 13 eBook: 978-0-7684-5627-1

ISBN 13 HC: 978-0-7684-5629-5

ISBN 13 LP: 978-0-7684-5628-8

For Worldwide Distribution, Printed in the U.S.A.

1 2 3 4 5 6 7 8 / 24 23 22 21 20

Important Notice

Dedication

I dedicate this book to the Lord my God who is my defense, my strong tower, my rock, my deliverer, and the God that heals. I will spend the rest of my days helping Your creation experience abundant health.

Contents

Faith Is a Place

A song of faith and hope
by Michael Neale and Jordan Rubin

VERSE 1

This shell that I've been livin' in
Is only temporary skin
There is so much more here
Than meets the eye
Through my body's prison bars
And out beyond the painful scars
I see a light, shining where you are
In my heart I run away
Break the chains of earthly fate
I know that I'll be whole again someday.

CHORUS

Faith is a place that I can go
In my heart and in my soul
I believe
Faith is the rock on which I stand
When I cannot see Your hand
I still believe.

VERSE 2

Outside broken down to dust
Inside I know who to trust
I know You will meet me when I run to You
Life is in Your grand design
I know You're not done with mine
So I will keep on running toward the light
Though I do not understand
The many facets of Your plan
I realize I'm safe inside Your hand.

CHORUS

Faith is a place that I can go
In my heart and in my soul
I believe
Faith is the rock on which I stand
When I cannot see Your hand
I still believe.

BRIDGE

I know You won't leave me here
You're acquainted with my tears
Somehow I just know a brighter day is near.

CHORUS

Faith is a place that I can go
In my heart and in my soul
I believe
Faith is the rock on which I stand
When I cannot see Your hand
I still believe
In faith.

Foreword

BY CHARLES STANLEY

Senior Pastor of First Baptist Church in Atlanta, Georgia
Founder and President of In Touch Ministries

JORDAN RUBIN IS ON A MISSION FROM GOD TO CHANGE THE HEALTH OF this nation. When I was first presented with the manuscript for this book, I couldn't put it down. I had been praying for more than a year that God would lead me to a health plan that was based on the Bible and tested by science. *The Maker's Diet* is just that.

Jordan's journey from sickness to health is a true testament to the handiwork of a loving and compassionate God. God took Jordan through the valley, delivered him, and positioned him to impact lives across the nation. His one and only focus is to help deliver people from the bondage of sickness and disease into the promised land of health.

Our nation's health is at an all-time low. I am constantly asked to pray for people who are suffering terribly from cancer, heart disease, diabetes, arthritis, and so many other diseases. People that I love have lost their lives and many productive years to debilitating illnesses.

Perhaps by following the principles outlined in this book these conditions would have been different. I have personally followed the Maker's Diet and noticed immediate improvements in my health. To my surprise, the food is absolutely wonderful. In fact, Jordan, his wife, Nicki, and I have shared many meals in the past, and I believe that making my health a priority will allow me to fulfill my mission to preach the gospel to all the ends of the earth.

One thing that separates the Maker's Diet from all the other health programs I've read about and tried is its truly holistic approach to health. *The Maker's Diet* incorporates the four pillars of health—which are physical, spiritual, mental, and emotional. The physical health plan incorporates diet, nutrition, exercise, hygiene, and body therapies that emphasize the importance of living in a healthy environment. The message of spiritual health is very clear. Each of us needs to find purpose in our life. We were all created for a reason. We were created to accomplish great things. Our connection with the Creator and His supreme purpose

The Maker's Diet for our lives makes every day worth living. Our mental health is vitally important. The ability to control our thought life and focus on the tasks at hand can shape who we are. Our emotional health and stability are interrelated with each of the other three pillars. We all encounter stress on a daily basis. Our circumstances are not always ideal. Stress and circumstances do not determine who we are. Our ability to handle adversity defines us. The health principles outlined in *The Maker's Diet* can provide you with the framee work to achieve health physically, spiritually, mentally, and emotionally.

The Maker's Diet by Jordan Rubin has made a significant difference in my life. I urge you to pay close attention to the principles outlined in this book and share them with the ones you love.

May God bless you and your family with incredible health.

Introduction

BY JORDAN RUBIN

YOU HEAR THE ALARM SCREECHING IN YOUR EAR AS YOU PEER AT THE clock, one eye barely open, in disgust. Two "snooze alarms" later, you struggle out of bed, moving slowly and feeling achy, wondering why you feel as if you haven't slept at all.

While you brush your teeth, you look in the mirror and see what must be someone else's face looking back at you. The face is tired with light wrinkling. The beginnings of a double chin are accented by dark circles underneath bloodshot eyes glaring from the mirror image.

You grab your size 16 pants and wonder how, at only age thirty-seven, you are thirty pounds heavier than when you first got married. You go to your kids' rooms, wake them up, and help them get dressed. You head to the kitchen to prepare breakfast for them, sensing a twinge of guilt that it isn't particularly healthy—but then, you are not quite sure what is healthy. There is so much conflicting information regarding health these days.

Despite your promise to yourself that you would start feeding your children healthy foods, it hasn't happened yet. Your daughter is fifteen pounds overweight, and your younger son has attention deficit hyperactivity disorder and asthma. You've been secretly hoping they would grow out of their health problems, but your wait continues with no improvements. Even though your doctor tells you their health problems have nothing to do with what they eat, somehow you know better.

You prepare your kids' lunches, making sure they are chock-full of "healthy" carbohydrates such as fortified bread, a small bag of oven-baked potato chips, a fat-free cookie, and a boxed juice drink that says it's healthy—right next to the "10 percent real fruit juice" sticker.

Your out-of-breath husband runs into the kitchen, already talking on his smartphone. He grabs a Danish, mixes French vanilla creamer into his coffee, and kisses you on the cheek as he heads out the door. Looking at him, you don't feel quite as bad about the weight you've put on. He has you beat by five pounds.

You hurry your children out the door. Now it's time for your breakfast. You pour yourself a large coffee with the same nondairy French vanilla creamer, flavored with artificial sweetener, and spread margarine on a bagel. You remember to have some orange juice, which is made from a concentrate, of course. The label says it contains as much calcium as a glass of milk.

Then you receive a phone call. It's your mother, and she sounds upset. Her arthritis is acting up again, and she wants you to take her back to the doctor. Apparently, her new medication isn't working the way her doctor promised. She has been very dependent on you since your father died last year of a massive heart attack. He was only sixty years old.

If this story sounds a lot like yours, you are not alone. It seems the state of our health as a nation is worse than ever before. Today, two-thirds of American adults are overweight, and one of three adults are obese. The number of those who are extremely obese—at least 100 pounds overweight—has quadrupled since the 1980s.

The impact of being the fattest nation on Earth has ramifications across the board. Our seniors are suffering from diseases such as osteoporosis, Alzheimer's, and dementia. Too many of the elderly spend many fruitless years of their lives being cared for in assisted living facilities with very little mental or physical function.

Next up are the Baby Boomers—those born between 1946 and 1964. They are clearly the generation of widespread obesity, a health condition leading to diabetes, cancer, and heart disease. It seems that the main reason some Baby Boomers do not get cancer is because their lives have already been claimed by sudden heart attack.

Then there are the Millennials, the first generation of young people to suffer in alarming numbers from chronic degenerative and autoimmune diseases such as multiple sclerosis, lupus, chronic fatigue syndrome, Crohn's disease, Type I diabetes, and even Parkinson's disease. The rates of infertility are staggering, causing more and more young women to seek fertility specialists. Alcohol abuse is high. And the addiction to opioids—from prescription pain relievers to fentanyl—has created an "overdose crisis." The Centers for Disease Control and Prevention in 2019 said that more than 130 people die every day from an overdose.

Considering all this bad news, it seems our very existence as a species is threatened if we don't change—and change quickly. But I have some good news for you: we can change. We can redirect our own health destiny.

Twenty-five years ago, I found myself suffering from an incurable illness. An effective treatment plan escaped nearly seventy doctors. Yes, I felt hopeless. Yes, I was afraid. And yes, I felt deserted...but I wasn't alone.

From the depths of my despair I heard a still, small voice say to me, *Everything is going to be okay.* After visiting what seemed like every doctor on the planet and trying every "miracle" drug, "miracle" diet, and "miracle" supplement, I found myself tearing through the pages of the world's oldest, most sacred, and best-selling book—the Bible.

What I was looking for in God's Word was not purely spiritual. I was looking for answers to my many debilitating health problems. What I found was a great health plan—and the only health program I will need for the rest of my life. This ancient health program literally transformed the life of a seemingly hopeless twenty-year-old, and I believe the same principles can pull you out of the grip of disease and help you enter the Promised Land of health.

Read This Book If...

The Maker's Diet may dramatically change and improve your life if:

1. You want to avoid disease and live as healthy as possible with abundant energy and improved physical appearance.
2. You are suffering from disease, feel hopeless, and doubt if you will ever get well because all of the specialists you have seen offer no answers.

While I make no claims to offer you a "cure-all," I believe this book was inspired by God and that the practical protocol it contains can greatly improve your health. The Maker has given me a program for vibrant health based on His Word and the best available science, in that order. The health principles on which this program is based are essentially the same—yesterday, today, and forever. (See Hebrews 13:8.) You too can enjoy the robust health and freedom from disease by simply following the health plan designed by our Creator.

Remember, the consequences of your health choices will affect many more people than yourself. You owe it to yourself and everyone you care about to return to the Maker's Diet.

1

From Tragedy to Triumph: My Personal Journey from Sickness to Health

M OST OF US ENTER THIS WORLD WITH GREAT FANFARE, FEW PROBLEMS, and no serious health problems. Some of us start life with debilitating disease or a serious health condition, which is viewed as tragic and rightly so. I was born as healthy as can be in 1975, the first child of parents who believed in following natural health practices in their own lives.

My father, Herb, was a naturopathic physician and a chiropractor who made every effort to help his family live the healthy lifestyle he advocated in his practice. My mother, Phyllis, was so in tune with my father that she gave birth to me at home with the assistance of four naturopathic students in Portland, Oregon.

Growing up, I was given no potentially hazardous immunizations. We all ate "health foods," as they were called in the late '70s and early '80s. One time, when one of my friends came to our house and was offered a glass of rice milk and soy cheese, he said that he wished he had visited the local 7-Eleven first to get some food he "recognized."

I also grew up with a good understanding of the Bible because of the devotion of my parents, who attended a messianic Jewish congregation outside of Atlanta, where my family moved after my second birthday. Messianic Jews, otherwise known as "Jewish Christians," believe Jesus is the Messiah.

Throughout childhood and in high school, I was rarely ill—I took antibiotics less than five times. Because I had never been hospitalized, I had no idea what it was like to be in a medical health center or even a pediatrician's office.

I was happy kid, a good student, and very involved in my local messianic and church ministries.

At the age of seventeen—my parents had started me in school early—I went to Florida State University in Tallahassee, Florida, on an academic scholarship. My extracurricular activities included a spot on the FSU cheerleading squad, campus ministry, singing in a traveling vocal group, and serving as the chaplain of my fraternity.

Shattered Dreams

The summer after my freshman year at Florida State is when my excellent health took a real nosedive. The first signs of failing health were periodic feelings of extreme exhaustion, which occurred during a stint as a summer camp counselor. I had always enjoyed an abundant energy level, but I actually fell asleep while riding the bus with some of my camp kids, who kept calling out, "Jordan! Wake up!" My lack of energy was embarrassing and soon became a regular occurrence.

My liveliness never returned, and without warning I faced an onslaught of other health problems, including nausea, stomach cramps, painful mouth sores, and recurring diarrhea. Believing these were temporary symptoms, I followed through with my commitment to be a counselor at a camp four hours from home.

Primitive Bathrooms

Most people would consider it difficult to camp out in Florida's simmering summer heat, and they would be correct. My unending nausea made the outdoor experience virtually impossible.

The usual "camp chow" wasn't helping. I gulped down quarts of sugary iced tea and became well acquainted with the camp's primitive outdoor bathrooms. I literally ran to the bare toilet fifteen or twenty times daily; as a result, I lost twenty pounds in seven days!

Until that time, I had an iron stomach. When TV commercials played for digestive products, I used to wonder what it felt like to have heartburn or diarrhea. Suddenly, I knew the feeling. These symptoms of extreme sickness and fatigue forced me to abruptly leave the camp. A friend had to drive me home because I was too sick to drive myself.

To spare my mom and dad concern, I delivered an Academy Award performance to hide my illness. I didn't want them to block my return to college, scheduled for ten days later. If I can just hang on until school starts, everything will be fine, I thought. I just need to get back into the swing of things.

My parents didn't think my request to see our family physician was anything out of the ordinary. I visited our local family doctor and told him about my nausea, constant diarrhea, weight loss, and constant fatigue. I also said I felt like I had cottonmouth. He immediately tested for viruses, including AIDS. The tests all came back negative, which made sense, considering I had never had a blood transfusion or been sexually active. Finally, the doctor prescribed antibiotics and sent me home.

Lean and Mean—and Back in School

Back at Florida State University, the severe gastrointestinal problems continued although I took the antibiotics faithfully. I tried to ignore what was happening to my body, but the symptoms forced me to discontinue my extra-curricular activities, including cheerleading on the sidelines of Seminoles' football games. I was still active in my local college church ministry, but I quit the fraternity I had joined. I also stopped studying for my American College of Sports Medicine exam.

I dropped to 145 pounds from my normal 180 pounds, and I felt as if I was falling apart. Each night I suffered a 104-degree fever and got little sleep between endless trips to the bathroom.

My Father's Dietary Supplements

My parents had certainly noticed my weight loss, and my dad sent me a package that included acidophilus, aloe juice, digestive enzymes, fiber supplements, and other herbal and nutritional products. I made myself believe those products would help me get well.

That was my introduction to alternative medicine, which turned out to be like jumping on a hamster wheel. While alternative medicine and dietary treatments can sometimes be better options than taking certain medications, most diets and supplements tend to over-promise and under-deliver.

In spite of the natural supplements I was taking, my symptoms didn't improve. Even worse, I was continually hungry. Food seemed to go right through me. I usually stuck to my healthy diet until a friend who worked at a sorority kitchen would bring home leftovers. That sent any good intentions about eating healthy right out the window.

I lived with seven other guys in a house rental, and we never missed an opportunity to give each other a hard time. We had a central message board used for jokes, harassing messages, and sometimes constructive and hilarious criticism for one another. One of my best friends wrote me a message that accurately reflected my changing physical appearance: "Hey, Jordan, Pee Wee Herman called. He wants his body back!"

In the mid-'90s, that was a cruel jest for several reasons we won't get into here, but I laughed, determined to keep a good sense of humor.

Increased Concern

I struggled to attend classes, but I avoided telling my parents how ill I was because I didn't want to leave school. One day as I walked to my music class, my right hip cracked as if it had dislocated. That's when I started to realize that something was seriously wrong.

My gastrointestinal problems had become "systemic," which means the pain spread to my joints and other parts of my body. My right hip constantly popped out of its socket. I even suffered minor dislocations getting in and out of cars.

I tried different diets along with nutritional supplements after I learned the "cottonmouth" sensation in my mouth indicated oral thrush, caused by a fungus called Candida albicans. My father put me on an eating plan called the Specific Carbohydrate Diet, made popular by Elaine Gottschall, author of Breaking the Vicious Cycle, to help alleviate the thrush and the diarrhea.

Desperation and a Difficult Diet

Although the Specific Carbohydrate Diet reportedly helped some people relieve symptoms, it was difficult for me to follow—especially at college. Unfortunately, I didn't have the self-discipline to stay on such a rigorous diet for very long, and the Specific Carbohydrate Diet didn't relieve my symptoms.

Instead, bathrooms became my obsession. Every life decision hinged on this key question: Where's the nearest bathroom? My friends stopped inviting me on long drives or to activities in isolated locations. Although I prayed constantly and kept a positive attitude as much as I could, the symptoms refused to cooperate, and relentless misery began to overwhelm me.

I Took One Look And...

Finally, I admitted to my parents how sick I was, and they arranged a flight home for me the very next day. When I walked in, my father took one look at me and strode into action. He took my temperature—and was shocked to discover a reading of 105 degrees. He immediately dumped a load of ice into our bathtub and filled it with cold water. Then he helped me gingerly get into the bathtub packed with ice cubes. As I shivered in the ice water, confused and delirious, I didn't know what was happening, but I remember hearing Dad cry out, "My God, I don't want my son to die."

The cold bath seemed to stabilize me, but my fever remained so high that my parents decided they had to take me to the local hospital, a first for me. The next morning I was admitted to the hospital, hoping to receive a cure-all prescription so I could get back to school. Instead, my "visit" lasted two full weeks! Depression set in as I lay in bed with intravenous fluids and antibiotics going into each arm.

My body was so overridden by infection that inflammation set in. Doctors prescribed two highly toxic intravenous steroid medications and put me through every test imaginable. I received more X-rays in two weeks than most people receive in a lifetime. While radiologists scanned my upper and lower gastrointestinal tracts, I felt as if they were conducting deluxe tours of my gut with a GoPro camera!

The results weren't encouraging. The doctor diagnosed Crohn's disease, an abnormal inflammation of the small bowel and colon that causes the intestinal wall to thicken. As this disease progresses, eventually the bowel channel narrows and blocks the intestinal tract, robbing the body of its ability to absorb nutrients.

Caution: Nightmare Ahead

As an added complication, I also had duodenitis, an inflammation of the duodenum (the first part of the small intestine) that afflicts less than 1 percent of Crohn's disease patients. As a result, I was literally starving to death. I was put on total parenteral nutrition (TPN) to put nutrients directly into my bloodstream.

Infection and pain raged through my body while emotional chaos gripped my mind. I tried to cope with the diagnosis of Crohn's disease—incurable, I was told—as best I could. Little did I know that my nightmare was just beginning.

My doctor said I could expect to live a normal life except for the lifelong need for medication and "a few surgeries." I would be able to father children, but only if I switched medications during the process of conception.

Facing the Facts

Though I was not familiar with Crohn's disease, I soon learned that according to the disease's pattern, my future looked bleak. Crohn's victims experience progressive symptoms of abdominal pain, diarrhea, extreme weight loss, and sometimes premature death. I was told that medications would keep me alive, but I quickly discovered that their side effects were nearly as bad as the disease itself. Science knew of no cause or cure for Crohn's at the time, and my prognosis was very poor.

Dr. Burrill Crohn, a New York City gastroenterologist, discovered Crohn's disease in the 1930s. One of the most famous persons to be diagnosed with the disease was former President Dwight Eisenhower. These days, approximately 1.6 million Americans suffer from Crohn's disease, ulcerative colitis, or some form of inflammatory bowel disease (IBD), with 70,000 new cases each year. Diagnoses of inflammatory bowel disease have been increasing dramatically in the last decade.

In fact, an incredible 85 percent of Americans are afflicted with some kind of digestive problem today. About two out of every ten Americans have been diagnosed with irritable bowel syndrome. With the sales of heartburn medications booming, some experts predict Crohn's disease may eventually surpass ulcers as the number one digestive problem in the United States.

Embarrassed by my symptoms, I simply told my friends I was sick and avoided details. I desperately hoped to return to school. Naively, I thought the doctor's "magic bullet" prescriptions would make me well, but health by medication wasn't working. Upon my discharge, I graduated from intravenous drugs in the hospital to taking oral medications such as prednisone at home.

The first day I took the oral form of prednisone, the synthetic corticosteroid triggered hallucinations, causing me to cry uncontrollably. I also took mesalamine for symptoms of ulcerative colitis—my doctors wanted me to cover all the bases—and the antimicrobials Flagyl and Diflucan for the chronic thrush.

For good measure, the doctors also put me on ciprofloxacin (Cipro), the drug of choice for nonspecific bacterial infections. I topped off this medical cocktail with regular doses of Zantac for the searing heartburn caused by the other medications.

My Worst Nightmare

Despite all the medications, my condition failed to improve. I still rushed to the bathroom up to thirty times a day. Most of my stools were bloody, and the severity of the cramps made me want to bang my head against the wall. But if my days were rough, my nights were worse. The persistent nocturnal diarrhea produced chronic sleep deprivation.

My bathroom visits continued 24/7, occurring every forty-five minutes or so. Only rarely did I get more than an hour of unbroken sleep per night. As the months passed, I existed in a state of fatigue and exhaustion—and for good reason. I had an almost unheard-of serum iron level of 0 despite my daily iron injections.

Iron is an essential component of hemoglobin, the oxygen-carrying protein in the blood. My low serum levels of albumin indicated I was suffering from a severe wasting disease known as cachexia, as well as low immunity and rapid deterioration of all body tissues. My body wasn't absorbing nutrition, which meant I was slowly starving to death.

Host of Bacteria

My main problem was that my digestive system wasn't absorbing nutrients, a condition called "malabsorption syndrome." So many toxic drugs were being prescribed for me that their chemical interactions created even more problems than my disease. Taken together, what was happening was quite a shock for a nineteen-year-old who had never been hospitalized before.

Like many Americans, I did not understand how important the gastrointestinal tract or gut was for optimum health. The gastrointestinal system, an engineering marvel and a creative wonder, is home to a host of bacteria and other microorganisms, some good for the body and some pathogenic or "bad."

Scientific and medical research has shown that a proper balance between these intestinal bacteria is key to long-term health. Unfortunately, the modern American diet is like opening a candy store in the human gut. The bad bacteria love to feast on sugars, high-carbohydrates, and refined foods.

The final blow to my health was caused by this bacterial imbalance in my digestive system called dysbiosis. This is what led to the breakdown of my body's immune barrier.

A Walking Medical Encyclopedia

Cutting-edge medical researchers now believe that life and death begin in the digestive tract. If your digestive system breaks down, you will likely encounter a host of seemingly unrelated but debilitating illnesses. In the following chart, I have listed the disease conditions that were working in my body:

MY PERSONAL DISEASE PROFILE

- *Chronic candidiasis* (or yeast overgrowth): I had the highest level possible.
- *Entamoeba histolytica*, a parasite that causes amebic dysentery
- *Cryptosporidiosis*, a protozoan infection that causes severe intestinal illness
- *Incipient diabetes* (my lower leg was purple because of extremely poor circulation)
- *Jaundice* (plus other liver and gallbladder problems that afflicted me)
- *Insomnia*
- *Hair loss*
- *Endocarditis*, a heart infection
- *Eye inflammation*
- *Prostate and bladder infections*
- *Extreme anemia* (my serum ferritin [iron] level was 0 for over twelve consecutive months)
- *Chronic electrolyte imbalance* (due to my constant dehydration)
- *Elevated C-reactive protein* (which indicated chronic inflammation and bacterial infection and increased my risk of heart attack and stroke)
- *Anemia,* or a shortage of red blood cells in the bloodstream (only red blood cells carry oxygen to muscle tissues and organs)
- *Chronic fatigue,* a mysterious ailment that includes symptoms of unceasing fatigue, headaches, weakness, aching muscles and joints, and the inability to concentrate

- *Arthritis,* which was marked by joint inflammation, stiffness, and pain (my immune system was mistakenly attacking itself; Crohn's disease is thought by some to be autoimmune in origin)
- *Leukocytosis,* an abnormal increase in white blood cells, especially immature cells
- *Malabsorption syndrome* (my body was unable to absorb sufficient nutrients from food, so no matter how much I ate, I was still starving)

My health worsened despite the treatments I received in the hospital. My ability to participate in any of life's activities totally stopped, which was quite a blow. I was used to being the ringleader who gathered people together. Instead, I had to tell my friends, "No, I can't come" or "No, I really can't do that."

I felt bad for my friends who called and wanted to visit. I felt I disappointed them, along with my parents, my sister, and my grandparents. They were all suffering as a result of my illness, and realizing that filled me with feelings of guilt.

FAMILY MEMBERS SUFFER, TOO
by
Jenna Rubin

"Where's my brother?"

"Oh, he's in the nurse's office. He's not feeling well. His stomach is bothering him."

The summer camp that I was attending had just begun. Jordan was a counselor at the camp, and I was just entering my teens. But I rarely saw him around camp because he spent so much time at the nurse's office.

Turns out he was really sick. I was upset over the whole thing, but no one knew any details about his symptoms. When he didn't get any better, Jordan had to go home early, leaving me behind.

At the start of camp, Jordan looked very healthy. He was really muscular, though he had gained some extra weight from eating junk food while away at college. By the end of the first week, though, he'd lost nearly twenty pounds. He didn't get better, and then when he returned to college, things got even worse. He got so sick that he had to come home.

I was in a rebellious stage at the time, so the combination of worry over Jordan and the big change in our lives triggered hidden anger in me. I loved Jordan, and I was really concerned about his health, but I came to the point where I couldn't believe he would ever get better.

Jordan didn't mean for this to happen, but his sickness essentially took my mother from me. She was always caring for him and trying to find another cure or another doctor somewhere. All of us felt frustration from not being able to do anything to help Jordan.

As my brother became sicker and more emaciated, people became uncomfortable around him. Yet, even in that difficult time, Jordan still had faith that God would one day heal him. I still remember him telling me over and over again how helpless he felt. He looked like a twig, and his hair was falling out in clumps. That was horrible to see.

I'll always remember the time Jordan blacked out in the kitchen and fell face forward toward the floor. I somehow caught him before he cracked his head open. His health really nosedived, so much so that he needed a wheelchair to get around the house.

Self-centeredness comes easy when you suffer from a debilitating disease, but it also bothered me to think about how much I was disappointing others. I tried to keep a positive attitude with my friends, but it was hard to express joy when pain continually pierced my stomach and joints. It was like experiencing the pain of a twenty-four-hour stomach virus or a bad case of food poisoning day and night with no end in sight.

Though I held to my faith that God would heal me, I was desperate enough to try anything. In those days before Google and various medical websites, I grasped at every piece of health literature, booklet, or magazine article just in case they contained the answers to my problem.

According to all of the information I was reading, my body's healing response had been "turned off" or compromised in some way. My hope was that some natural method would help reactivate it.

My father joined me in the search for natural pathways to renewed health, and this became our shared obsession. Ultimately, our search took me to seventy health practitioners from seven different countries and a wide variety of medical doctors, naturopaths, chiropractors, immunologists, acuuncturists, homeopaths, herbalists, colon therapists, nutritionists, and dieticians.

None could pinpoint a reason for why I became so sick. Only God knows why I got sick, but looking back, the most probable culprit was my changed diet and lifestyle during my first year in college. College life brought a whole new stress level to my existence, much of it generated by my over-commitment of time. And in my quest for being in tip-top shape for the cheerleading squad, I adopted a diet that was very high in carbohydrates (mostly from processed grains, dairy, and sugar) and dangerously low in fat and protein.

The hard truth is that my college diet was tailor-made for inducing the symptoms of most diseases, especially digestive illnesses.

One More Try

Despite my disappointing experience with the Specific Carbohydrate Diet, I still believed that staying on it without deviations would help me, so I tried the special diet one more time.

Dad arranged things so that I could consult daily on the phone with Elaine Gottschall, author of Breaking the Vicious Cycle. She had worked with a phyksician, Dr. Sydney Haas, to heal her daughter of ulcerative colitis, a disease very similar to Crohn's disease. Despite my fanatical adherence to the Specific Carbohydrate Diet for three to six months on three different occasions, the health plan didn't work for me.

This roadblock led to personal consultations with some of the foremost practitioners and diet experts in the world. I was a patient of Dr. Robert Atkins, author of The Atkins Diet. I met with Barry Sears, Ph.D., author of the best-selling health book, The Zone. I consulted with Jeffrey Bland, Ph.D., a highly regarded functional medicine expert who put me through several rounds of his detoxification/elimination diet.

Nothing worked, even though these health professionals were extremely knowledgeable, highly educated, and quite sincere about wanting to help me. Each of their diets had solid underpinnings, but something was missing.

During a two-year search for a cure, my father spent approximately $150,000 on natural health treatments for me, including thirty probiotic formulas, countless enzymes, fiber, anti-Candida and antiparasitic formulas, and numerous immune-boosting and detoxification products. He had to borrow against our house to pay for everything, but that's how much he and Mom were willing to see me returned to good health.

Running the Gamut

Why did I put myself through such difficult and expensive regimens? That's easy to answer: I wanted to get better and end the pain. Those were powerful motivators.

I tried everything and did anything. When someone said my liver was the problem, I decided to detoxify my liver. That didn't work. When one "health expert" from the United Kingdom said he had cured 250 patients with Crohn's disease, I agreed to undergo cell therapy with injectable sheep cells taken from embryos. The needles were huge, but, predictably, the results were nonexistent. I also tried retention enemas, colonics, and even more liver detoxification methods.

I tried taking "glandulars," or glandular and organ extracts taken from the dried tissues of every conceivable animal organ and gland. I even took adrenal cortical extract, or ACE, an extract of bovine adrenal glands thought to possess the powers of hydrocortisone, which had been used extensively in medicine.

For nearly a year, I injected myself seven times a day with vitamins and minerals, using a small needle reserved for insulin injections. I had become so emaciated that when I injected myself in the shoulders and the sides of my hips, I could feel the needle hitting bone.

Got Any Cabbage Juice and Shark Cartilage?

The list goes on.

When I read that cabbage juice was good for the gut and rich in organic sulfur compounds, I consumed large amounts of cabbage juice. I did the same with wheat grass juice, Chinese and Peruvian herbs, Japanese kampo, olive leaf extract, and shark cartilage. I tried the macrobiotic diet, the raw food vegan diet, and nitrogenated soy as well. So yummy....

My desperate hunt for a cure drove me to travel to clinics in Europe, South America, Mexico, and Canada—often in a wheelchair. Without exception, the doctors and health practitioners who treated me characterized my appearance as that of a concentration camp victim. Despite my fragile health, I endured the perils of traveling to alternative cancer clinics in Mexico and Germany, returning in worse condition than when I left.

Through it all, I drew strength from my faith in God's love for me. I was difficult to live with and at times my hope was dim, but God remained faithful.

The psalmist David expressed my pain and revived my hope during daily readings from Psalm 31:

> *In You, O Lord, I put my trust; Let me never be ashamed; Deliver me in Your righteousness. Bow down Your ear to me, Deliver me speedily; Be my rock of refuge, A fortress of defense to save me… I will be glad and rejoice in Your mercy, For You have considered my trouble; You have known my soul in adversities… Have mercy on me, O Lord,* **for I am in trouble***; My eye wastes away with grief, Yes, my soul and my body! For my life is spent with grief, And my years with sighing;* **My strength fails** *because of my iniquity,* **And my bones waste away***… I am forgotten* **like a dead man, out of mind***; I am like a broken vessel. But as for me, I trust in You, O Lord; I say, "You are my God."* **My times are in Your hand;** *Deliver me from the hand of my enemies, And from those who persecute me. Make Your face shine upon Your servant; Save me for Your mercies' sake.*
>
> —Psalm 31:1–2,7,9–10,12,14–16 NKJV
> (bold italics added for emphasis)

False Data Supplied by Scientists for Hire

As I grew more frantic, I tried almost five hundred different "miracle" products (including two or three treatments no rational person would consider). I knew what it meant to be desperate. I became the victim—and I choose that word carefully—of many network marketers and mass distributors of health products who made outrageous and unfounded health claims that contained little, if any, scientific substance.

My dad scoured health magazines and called colleagues around the world searching for clinics and therapies that might help. The many machines I hooked up to my body could have come out of a science fiction novel!

Weird Science

Some of the practitioners I visited performed various forms of electrodermal screening (EDS), a method of computerized information-gathering based on physics and acupuncture meridians.

After one doctor probed me with his EDS machine, he said my illness was due to electromagnetic fields in my house. I had to do something about that, so I slept in a steel cage placed around my bed. At night I was instructed to shut off the TV and clocks—and all electrical devices. In case you're wondering, that approach didn't work. The next EDS practitioner told me that I was having an adverse reaction from a certain orbiting satellite. This is what I call weird science from the outer reaches of the alternative health field.

But I also exhausted other areas of alternative medicine. I tried applied kinesiology, a type of chiropractic where different tests for muscle strength and weakness were done on points of my body. I utilized acupuncture and homeopathy but didn't find any relief. Taking various medications and supplements was my life.

When I wasn't visiting a doctor several times a week, I stayed at home in my chair and fantasized while watching cooking shows. That's when I felt like I developed a special bond with Chef Emeril on the Food Network back in his heyday.

I used all of my spare time puzzling over what products to use and what might help me, and I devoured more than three hundred health and nutrition books. I would locate well-known authors and arrange personal consultations, refusing to meet with anyone but the best.

But none of them had answers for me.

'Til There Was You

Most of the doctors and practitioners I visited said they could cure me in a short period of time. One after another assured me they had never failed to cure their patients, but they made promises they couldn't keep. Their claims to healing weren't totally unfounded, because most of them had anecdotal evidence based on patient testimony. Yet the results were not there for me.

Like many others who are desperately ill, I was willing to believe and put my faith in these medical practitioners. Seeing them was difficult, though. My frequent bladder and eye infections made it extremely unsettling to travel, but I hauled my decaying body to their offices anyway in hope of finding a cure.

Here's how bad things got. One time, while waiting for an airplane to take off, I calmly said to myself, "If this plane went down, that wouldn't be a bad thing." That was my mental state during the darkest days of my desperate journey. I was not suicidal, but I felt so hopeless. I just couldn't handle the pain anymore.

I wasn't actively seeking death, but I reasoned that if I died, then at least I could join my Creator and be pain-free. Again, it was the psalmist who perfectly expressed my feelings at that point:

I am troubled, I am bowed down greatly; I go mourning all the day long. For my loins are full of inflammation, And there is no soundness in my flesh. I am feeble and severely broken; I groan because of the turmoil of my heart...My heart pants, my strength fails me; As for the light of my eyes, it also has gone from me...For in You, O Lord, I hope; You will hear, O Lord my God.

—Psalm 38:6–8, 10, 15 (NKJV)

A last ray of hope drew me to Germany to receive an experimental drug made from the juices of the Venus flytrap plant. At that time the U.S. Food and Drug Administration did not permit this herbal substance to be imported, so that meant making the long flight across the Atlantic Ocean.

My Big Fat German Nightmare

My mother accompanied me to Germany. It was a twenty-eight-hour nightmare involving numerous planes, trains, but no automobiles.

Upon landing Frankfurt, we missed one train because my mom and I couldn't drag our luggage fast enough, so we had to wait six hours for the next departure. I passed the time by locating and frequently visiting the public bathroom, which smelled and wasn't clean.

Upon arrival at the medical clinic, my German doctor instructed me to discontinue my medications, including prednisone, which I had been taking for over a year. I suffered devastating withdrawal symptoms, including an inability to catch my breath for three days. My German doctor concluded that my problem rested with my immune system. He said certain parts were overactive and others were underactive.

After my mother left—she had to return to her job as a schoolteacher because of the financial pressures—I stayed alone in the clinic for six long weeks. While I was in the hands of sadly inattentive doctors and nurses, none of their therapies produced positive results.

Mental Problem or Doctor Problem?

After six weeks going nowhere, my doctor egotistically announced that I wasn't getting well because I had "mental problems."

Think about what this did for my fragile psyche. I was a nineteen-year-old forced by a life-threatening illness to drop out of college and abandon my dreams. I was separated from my family and friends by thousands of miles and the Atlantic Ocean. I was trapped in a German health clinic where no one spoke English; the ceiling of my room was less than five feet high (ouch!); and most of the people assigned to my care seemed to view me more as a nuisance than as a patient. Considering that combination, I suppose such an isolated existence could produce mental problems in anyone.

Miserable and in constant pain, I felt imprisoned in my own body. A cloud of despair covered me. Would I ever enjoy a normal life again? Would I ever sleep through the night or wake up without pain? Would I ever be healthy again?

It was time to go home, but soon I discovered that making the trip was easier said than done. With great difficulty, I checked myself out and waited for a cab to take me to the airport with my luggage.

I was so frail that the taxi driver had to help me into the back of his cab.

Stranded in Germany

Upon arrival at the airport curb, my driver got someone with a wheelchair since I was too weak to walk unassisted to the check-in counter. None of the airline employees at the ticket counter understood English, and they couldn't find any record of my ticket. Knowing I couldn't go back to the clinic—and having nowhere to go—I offered to purchase another ticket with my credit card, but the transaction was declined by my credit card company.

That did it. My life had spiraled out of control at the ticket counter, complicated by a painful urinary tract infection and pinkeye in both eyes, along with my chronic bowel problems. It seemed like I was out of options. It appeared I wouldn't get home.

In extreme desperation, I quickly prayed: Lord, I cannot do a single thing. I am putting my life in Your hands. Please help me get out of this situation. I feel completely hopeless.

Within minutes, a gate agent made a startling discovery—she found my reservation in her system. My ticket was printed out, and I boarded the plane.

Though I missed my connecting flight in New York, I finally made it to the West Palm Beach airport after a thirty-hour ordeal. I cannot describe how relieved I was to be home.

Shortly afterward, I was hospitalized a second time, completely dehydrated with a resting heart rate of 200–260 beats per minute. I couldn't even keep water down, and I weighed only 104 pounds.

I was skin and bones, wasting away and near death.

At Death's Door

My veins were so dry and tapped out that it took a team of nurses and doctors two and one-half hours to insert an IV into my right arm. I overheard one of the nurses say to another health-care giver, "That poor boy isn't going to make it through the night."

Hopelessness flooded my being, and all I could do was pray. At that point, I was ready to go home and be with my Creator. Though I felt I had lived an incredible life for someone my young age, I was disappointed that I had never fallen in love, gotten married, and had children. In spite of my pain, I thanked my Creator for a wonderful life, committed myself into His hands, and mentally prepared myself to die.

I drifted into a fitful sleep and awoke to see my grandmother leaning over me with her hand on my forehead. Several nurses entered to announce that they had managed to get a blood return and could hook me up to another IV. Then I was helped out of bed to stand on a scale. Great news! I had gained ten pounds of water weight in one night. I felt a new resolve shiver throughout my body. I was going to make it. I was sure of it.

At last, a glimmer of real hope—that is, until the doctors prescribed the same medications I had been given during my first hospital stay. Once again, I became a human drugstore filled with antibiotics, antifungals, antiparasitics, heartburn medications, and prednisone. When I finally left the hospital and the doctors switched me from intravenous to oral medications, I experienced hallucinations once again.

In the words of baseball's Yogi Berra, "It was déjà vu all over again."

Picturing Such a Pathetic Sight

Despite everything I had been through, including hundreds of unfulfilled promises by doctors and health practitioners, I still clung to the hope that God would deliver me.

One morning, while still bedridden, I made a request to my mother. "Mom, I want you to take a picture of me," I said. My unusual request completely startled her.

"Why in the world do you want me to take a picture of you?" she replied.

With all the courage I could muster, I softly answered, "Because no one will believe me when I get well. No one will ever believe that I was this sick. I'm getting out of bed, and I need you to take my picture."

I nearly fell going from my bed to the hallway, and Mom needed to hold my elbow to get me there, but we got the picture. All of my options seemed to be exhausted the day my mother snapped that photo. The reason I had a beard at the time was because I was too weak to shave and couldn't afford to cut myself with my unsteady hand.

Two Terrible Choices

The day Mom shot that picture, I weighed a whopping 111 pounds, but my body was wasting away and my future still looked bleak. One doctor told me that my only hope was to travel to Mount Sinai Hospital in New York City for the removal of my large intestines and part of my small intestines. Or, my only other alternative was a J-Pouch operation, which is the surgical removal of the colon followed by the construction of an internal pouch to collect the body's solid waste.

Faced with two terrible choices balanced against a lifetime of unrelenting pain or death, I reluctantly decided with my family to go to Mount Sinai and get whatever surgery I needed. My primary physician called my condition "the worst case of Crohn's disease" he had ever seen. He doubted I would live long enough to return home.

That revelation forced me to reexamine my options. The multiple medications I was prescribed only made me feel worse, but there was always the chance they'd work and my ill effects would be reversed. The problem with surgery was its permanence.

The other consideration was that I had only a little bit of fight left, so I didn't want to waste what little energy I had by going under the knife.

A Final Ray of Hope

Shortly after I was wheeled out of the hospital early in 1996—still not cured, still no better than before—my father took it upon himself to contact Bud Keith, an eccentric nutritionist in San Diego, after investigating the man's nutritional program. He didn't tell me what he was doing because the last thing my father wanted to do was get my hopes up prematurely.

Bud Keith said he believed I was ill because I was not eating the diet of the Bible. The nutritionist based the failure of the doctors who treated me on the fact that they did not base their treatments upon biblical principles.

What he said made me curious, so I decided to ditch the idea of surgery and fly out to San Diego to give this so-called Bible diet a try. What did I have to lose? In fact, I doubled down and stopped taking all nutritional products.

Before I left Florida, I studied what people ate thousands of years ago in the Bible. My studies uncovered an interesting fact: these ancient cultures consumed "living" foods that abounded with nutrients, enzymes, and beneficial microorganisms as well as healthy animal foods that were rich in nutrients. There were no processed foods thousands of years ago, so they weren't consuming "empty" calories that robbed nutrients from the body.

Feeling like I was on to something, I was excited to fly out to San Diego so that Bud Keith could teach me how to eat "God's way." I was so weak that I needed to be pushed on and off my flights with a wheelchair. But I knew I should live closer to this man and learn all that I could about turning my health around.

I'm glad I did. For the first time in my long battle, I saw some improvement in my health after integrating the nutritionist's program with my own findings about nutrition and health from the Bible.

A Bag of Black Powder

While I was in San Diego, my father decided to send me a plastic bag containing a black-colored powder. (Although he had promised not to send me any other nutritional products, he couldn't help himself.) He said it was a special type of probiotic or friendly bacteria.

Unfortunately, I had already tried thirty different varieties of probiotics with no success. How would this one be any different? How could my father expect me to eat this? It looked like dirt! Dad called to encourage me anyway, saying, "It may look like dirt, but it isn't. This substance contains healthy compounds from the soil."

An article enclosed with the package explained that these nutrients were missing from today's pesticide-sterilized, barren soils. The newsletter story claimed that the contents of the bag contained far more than trace minerals—it contained vital organisms that were called soil-based organisms, or SBOs. These friendly microorganisms have been largely wiped out by the pesticides, herbicides, fungicides, and synthetic fertilizers used on America's farm lands, by pasteurization, and by modern man's disdain for all microorganisms—even those life-supportive "bugs" or microscopic organisms our bodies need for maximum health.

All of the health research that I had read up to that point validated the fact that our soil is extremely deficient. It made sense that deficient soil leads to deficient bodies. After trying several hundred different "miracle" nutritional products, though, I was understandably jaded.

But for some reason this black powder was different.

Adding to My Diet

Having nothing to lose, I decided to include the odd-looking dirt organisms in my daily diet. I also added other items to my "biblical" diet, such as:

* kefir, which is a naturally fermented beverage made from raw goat's and cow's milk
* organically raised, free-range, or grass-fed meats
* eggs and meat from healthy chickens
* ocean-caught wild fish
* natural sprouted or sourdough breads made from yeast-free whole grains
* raw nuts and seeds
* organic fruits and vegetables
* raw sauerkraut
* carrot and other vegetable juices

These "live" foods were filled with beneficial enzymes, vitamins, minerals, and friendly microorganisms.

My health didn't reappear magically in one day; it takes time to overcome years of illness. I actually felt a little worse for the first thirty days as my body purged itself of lingering toxins. The nausea increased slightly, my digestion got a little worse, and my energy levels dropped lower than usual. But I felt like I was on the right track.

I was experiencing a Herxheimer reaction, or the "die-off" effect that many people experience when they dramatically improve their diet and lifestyles. It is an allergic response to the toxic byproducts produced when the body's pH is changed for the better, causing large numbers of pathological organisms, such as harmful bacteria and yeast organisms, to die and exit the body.

The collective effect of this reaction is a temporary worsening of symptoms, and I was aware that was a possibility. In reality, what was happening to my body was an indication that I was responding positively to treatment. Significant improvement would follow this initial detoxification reaction.

Since the time of Hippocrates, it's been understood that the symptoms of most diseases represent the efforts of the body to eliminate toxins. Gradually for me, a newfound energy emerged, and I visited the bathroom less frequently. One month after I added the black powder to my diet, I noticed a marked improvement in my overall health.

Becoming Something of a Bum

After I landed in San Diego, I purchased a used motor home so I could stay close to the beach and breathe the ocean air. I became something of a beach bum for forty days and nights as I tried to find places to park at night where I wouldn't get fined, towed away, or arrested. Living on the streets—twenty-five years before homelessness became a national crisis—was an unusual experience for a kid from the suburbs.

Different friends flew out from Florida to help me, and I spent each day praying, listening to music, and planning the preparation of my daily medicine—my food. Amazingly, after my two brutal years of suffering, I gained twenty-nine pounds during those forty days, reaching an incredible (for me) weight of 151 pounds!

On my twenty-first birthday, my buddy Jason Dewberry took an "after" photograph on the beach—four months after I arrived in California. I wasn't completely well at that point, but I was on my way to full recovery. I weighed 170 pounds and felt like the happiest man in the world.

Psalm 30, which I had prayed for so long, was coming to pass. I encourage you to read the entire psalm, but I am including some important verses here:

> *I will extol You, O Lord; for You have lifted me up And have not let my foes to rejoice over me. O Lord my God, I cried unto You, And You healed me. O Lord, You brought up my soul from the grave: You have kept me alive, that I should not go down to the pit.... You have turned for me my mourning into dancing; You have put off my sackcloth and clothed me with gladness To the end that my glory may sing praise to You and not be silent. O Lord my God, I will give thanks to You forever.*
>
> —PSALM 30:1–3, 11–12 (NKJV)

God worked a miracle in my life. The combination of the biblical diet and the unique soil organisms known as SBOs restored my health! I gained more than fifty pounds in three months. By December 1996, after two years of hopeless suffering, I was back home in Florida—fully restored and ready to start my life again. Praise God!

By the grace of God, I had done what millions of disease victims desperately hope to do—I had conquered illness and recovered my health.

LIKE A BODYBUILDER
by
Jenna Rubin

After Jordan decided to go to California to work with a man who claimed his Bible-based diet would help him, he told us in phone calls that he was feeling better and gaining weight. Three months into his program, Mom and I flew to San Diego to see him, and we were thrilled to see him standing on his own. We were so excited!

He was still thin, and you could tell that he wasn't perfectly healthy—but he was getting better. His hair was still thin and weird looking, but it was starting to grow back.

There are two things I remember the most about seeing Jordan in San Diego. First, his attitude was really positive, something missing back in Florida. The second thing happened at the beach when he insisted on picking me up and carrying me around like some Venice Beach bodybuilder. That's when I knew Jordan's strength was definitely coming back, which filled us all with hope.

≈

FROM PEE WEE HERMAN TO BEST MAN
by Jason Dewberry

"Hey, Jordan, Pee-wee Herman called. He wants his body back!"

When I wrote this quip on our message board in our rental house near the Florida State campus in Tallahassee, none of us who lived with Jordan knew how close he would come to death over the next year.

As one of Jordan's closest friends—we were inseparable at Palm Beach Gardens High—I witnessed his painful destruction from a front-row seat. Growing up, I was one of the friends who used to rummage through the Rubins' kitchen in bewilderment. Even to this day, I don't know how you get milk from rice.

I watched Jordan struggle with this mysterious sickness, and I saw this extremely active and athletic guy begin to wear down in unexplained exhaustion and lose his zest for life. As Jordan's condition started to progress further, I became unusually alarmed.

Jordan embodied what I thought was the ultimate health-conscious individual with a basically healthy diet, plenty of exercise, a clean lifestyle, and a positive attitude.

Throughout his entire high school and brief college life, he didn't consume a single alcoholic beverage or partake in any recreational drugs, and he practiced sexual abstinence due to his spiritual beliefs. To see him literally waste away before my eyes was very, very difficult.

We had been very involved in activities at church together, and I became his main contact with friends for updates on Jordan's condition. After a long period of trying to dispense hope to them, I found it hard to give any good news—because there just wasn't any.

My best friend was wasting away and dying, and there was nothing anyone could do about it. Some days I would wake up crying, thinking to myself, *This is it. I'm going to lose my best friend.*

One Thanksgiving holiday in the middle of Jordan's darkest time, I decided to read a letter at church that he had written to me in which he declared that he would be healed by faith.

He quoted a powerful Bible verse from Hebrews 11:1: *"Faith is the substance of things hoped for, the evidence of things not seen."*

Jordan believed that true faith could be proclaimed only during the midst of the storm, not in retrospect.

Things got so bad that one time when I walked into his house, I saw him in such an emaciated state that I almost threw up—not out of revulsion but out of fear.

How can this person still be alive? I asked myself. *One of his legs is thinner than my wrist!*

I felt an intense, gripping, emotional fear that this person who had so much to give, whose love was so infectious, was sitting in front of me looking as if he had just been liberated from a concentration camp.

Even though it was difficult to be around him, I wouldn't leave his side. There were times when Jordan would ask the why questions, but 90 percent of the time he was saying, "I'm going to keep my faith. When I get through this, when God heals me, He is going to use me to accomplish great things. I know He has a plan for my life."

No wonder that one of Jordan's favorite Bible verses was Jeremiah 29:11: "'For I know the plans I have for you,' declares the Lord, 'plans to prosper you and not to harm you, plans to give you hope and a future'" (NIV).

I just couldn't understand that. I had to come full circle and witness everything that happened in his life to see that Jordan was right. He had a genuine vision from God, and he knew he would be in front of people one day telling his story.

When Jordan went to San Diego, he asked me to come and help. That "after picture" of Jordan, which has now been seen by millions of people, was taken at Pacific Beach in front of Crystal Pier. Every morning after we drove to Boney's, a local health food store, to get raw kefir and raw cheeses, we parked our RV only fifty yards away from Crystal Pier. We would have cheeseburgers for breakfast—you know, organic cheeseburgers with wholegrain buns.

He was thrilled to have some semblance of his life back, and I was thrilled to have my old friend back. I was with him the night he proposed to his wife, Nicki, and I was the best man in his wedding. I was with him when he brought his first child home from the hospital. Now I have the opportunity to describe what God can do in one man's life when that person yields to His will.

Some Doctors Were Excited, Most Were Skeptical

I immediately told many of the doctors who had treated me about my dramatic recovery and even mailed them my "before" and "after" pictures, fully confident they would all be eager to learn about the regimen that had healed me. Some of them were excited, but most were skeptical.

Dr. Morton Walker, a medical journalist who had supplied me information on some of the clinics I visited, asked if he could write an article outlining my amazing story. He published the article in the Townsend Letter for Doctors and Patients, an alternative health publication that focuses on alternative medeicine and treatments. In those pre-Internet days, the article generated over 2,000 phone calls from doctors and individuals who wanted to try the Maker's Diet along with the SBOs.

Overnight, I decided to find a way to distribute the SBOs that had helped me get well, which led me to found a health and wellness company. I also went on to earn advanced degrees in nutrition and sports medicine and continued my studies for doctoral degrees in naturopathy and nutrition.

"MOM, I'M GOING TO GET WELL"
by
Phyllis Rubin

No mother should have to see her vibrant, athletic, college-age son fitted for a wheelchair, but I did. At six feet, one inch and 180 pounds, Jordan was in incredible shape and on fire for God. He was full of energy and loved life—until he got very sick. After a series of antibiotics, Jordan went back to college weighing 150 pounds. Before long, he showed up at our door weighing only 135 pounds with a 105-degree fever!

My husband and I looked at Jordan and thought, *My goodness, what is wrong with our son?* He wasn't the same person. He could barely walk, and many times he'd faint just walking to the bathroom. No one was able to diagnose Jordan until we found a doctor familiar with his symptoms.

He looked at Jordan and immediately said, "Your son has Crohn's disease."

Jordan's health went downhill from there. He progressively got sicker and lost more weight, and his hair began falling out. It was a mother's worst nightmare. We tried many doctors, drugs, and natural therapies; nothing seemed to work. I remember when Jordan had his first upper GI series. As he walked to the X-ray room looking like a very sick old man, he fainted and fell to the floor.

Later, toward the end when we really thought we might lose him, Jordan asked me to take his picture. It was hard to even look at him, much less take a picture of him. I wanted to tell him, "Don't wear shorts." It hurt me to see his bony legs and joints—he was just skin and bones. A few of my friends told me, "You have to let him go."

I'm not a negative person, but it was hard to watch my effervescent son have the life sucked out of him. I just cried my eyes out and kept praying for a miracle. When I traveled to Germany with him to seek treatment, I remember weeping after I dropped him off at the clinic. I prayed, "Lord, take care of my son; he's in Your hands. I give him to You, Lord. I have no other choice." It was one of the most difficult and greatest things I've ever done.

It was just a few months later that Jordan tried a primitive version of what he now calls the Maker's Diet for one week. I will never forget the day he smiled and told me, "Mom, I'm going to get well!" This was the first time I remember Jordan smiling in over a year. On that momentous day Jordan was right—and God was faithful!

Discovering Divine Destiny

My mission in life since my recovery has been to help sick and ill people regain their health and to help the healthy folks flourish even more. It seems obvious to me that I endured my ordeal for a reason—to discover a major part of the divine destiny for my life. I can't believe that I've been able to help so many people in the last twenty-five years.

These days, I believe I can speak with authority on nutrition, disease, and health not because I have paid my dues but because I have personally survived the tortuous walk through the valley of disease and death and emerged triumphant.

With this timely revision of *The Maker's Diet*, I've been enjoying good health and have been free of symptoms and medications since 1996. They say that Crohn's disease is supposedly incurable. Because of my experience, I can confirm that no disease is incurable.

Although the disease process in some people may be too advanced for them to recover completely, I am convinced that every person's state of health can be greatly improved. By following biblically and historically proven health principles, an individual can return to a diet and lifestyle that will lead to regeneration of the entire body, mind, soul, and spirit.

I remember my darkest days and telling myself that if I can help just one person who is suffering to overcome his or her illness, then it will have been worth it. When I was cured, I dedicated my life to teaching others how to attain the level of health and wellness they can only dream of, and I've stayed true to that promise.

My experiences also taught me a very important truth: the best way to cure disease is to never get it. I believe that everyone, whether presently healthy or ill, can benefit by incorporating the principles of the Maker's Diet into their lives.

This program is for you whether you want to avoid disease, enjoy a long and healthy life, overcome the painful symptoms of illness, lose twenty pounds, or prevent a disease that runs in your family.

My bout with severe illness made me a stronger person. I can relate to the biblical character Job, who suffered severe loss and extreme illness before God restored his health and increased his fortunes. The Lord has restored to me what was taken away, and He has multiplied it more than I could have ever asked or imagined.

Many would say that my healing and restoration began when I discovered the diet and health secrets of the Great Physician as followed by the world's healthiest people. I believe the spark that ignited the flame of healing in my life was the faith that God allowed my illness for a reason, and if I would trust Him, He would restore my health and direct my path.

Today, more than fifteen years after the release of *The Maker's Diet*, I'm still on a mission from God to change people's lives and give you a message of hope and healing. I will spend the rest of my life telling the world the truth that will set you free.

> *I waited patiently for the Lord; And He inclined unto me, And heard my cry. He also brought me up out of a horrible pit, Out of the miry clay, And set my feet upon a rock, And established my steps. He has put a new song in my mouth— Praise to our God; Many will see it and fear, And will trust in the Lord.*
>
> —Psalm 40:1–3 (NKJV)

2

The World's Healthiest People

THERE WAS A TIME WHEN MANY AMERICANS ASSUMED THAT THE United States was the world's healthiest nation. That may have been true when America landed the first astronauts on the moon, but those days are long gone. Unfortunately, all you have to do is study today's statistics for obesity—or look around a public place like a shopping mall—to understand that we are not as healthy as we may think.

We do enjoy one of the highest standards of living in the world, coupled with extraordinary emergency medical technology and trauma care. While Washington goes back and forth on the future of our health care system, Americans, for the most part, have access to excellent health care, but this fact doesn't make us healthy. Too many people end up in the emergency room these days, not because they had an accident but because they experienced a significant, life-threatening condition like a heart attack or a stroke.

It's during those moments that people experience a wake-up call about their health, which is quite different than pursuing a lifestyle that prevents disease. The concept of preventative medicine deserves much more attention than the lip service it currently receives, especially in the mainstream media.

The influence of advertising is a major reason why most Americans eat great quantities of food frequently, based on convenience. In fact, the entire fast food and TV dinner industries have flourished due to our fast-paced lifestyles that demand we eat "convenient" foods that can be prepared quickly—either at a drive-thru restaurant or out of a microwave oven. A recent phenomenon is food-delivery services like Home Chef, HelloFresh, and EveryPlate, which can be a great start in the right direction, but they are expensive for what arrives at your front door in a delivery box.

Unfortunately, the Creator didn't design our bodies to operate at optimum levels on fast food, junk food, or prepackaged foods. His laws still govern our entire human nature, including our health, and they bring consequences when violated, whether or not we accept the argument that they are still in place.

Elmer A. Josephson, a pioneer who dared to challenge the stream of popular dietary trends, had this to say in his book, God's Key to Health and Happiness:

> There is no portion of the commandments of God in general, or
> of the Mosaic code in particular, that is not based on a scientific
> understanding of fundamental law. The laws of God are enforced
> and are as sure as the law of gravity.

All of God's laws are like His law of gravity—and they cannot be changed. Our Creator specifically designed our bodies to function best on the Maker's Diet. In order to benefit from His plan, though, we must examine exactly what food is "biblical" and what food is unclean, unhealthy, or unacceptable according to both God and science—and in that order.

History reveals that the healthiest people in the world were generally the most primitive people as well. Our ancestors rarely died from the diet- and lifestyle-related illnesses that kill most modern people before their time. The reason they lived so healthy was because they ate healthier foods and had more active lifestyles. They foraged from "first level" food sources such as wild game, fresh-caught fish from the sea or inland waterways, wild berries, nuts, and plant foods.

Under these primitive hunter-gatherer conditions, food wasn't an afterthought; it was vital for survival. Primitive people "ate to live."

Contrast that to today, when we have allowed food to become our idol. Too many people admittedly "live to eat"—and look how "foodies" are celebrated as judges on cooking shows. Most modern men and women have strayed far from the Creator's foods, the same foods that have traditionally nourished the world's healthiest people. In our indiscriminating society, though, we say yes to virtually every whim and desire of our palate, resulting in a national dilemma of becoming overweight, sedentary, and increasingly sick.

The Top Five Diseases

The Top Five leading causes of hospitalization, according to a recent study by the Centers for Disease Control and Prevention, were diagnoses of:

* circulatory diseases (such as heart attacks)
* diabetes (which is usually related to obesity)
* diseases of the respiratory system (often cancer-related)
* diseases of the digestive systems (such as diverticulitis, peptic ulcers, and hemorrhoids)
* diseases of the genitourinary system (the reproductive organs and the urinary system)

These five classes represent diseases of lifestyle, revealing the hazardous effects of civilization, which are expanding as industrialization and modernization spread to more of the world's nations and cultural groups. These diseases are still uncommon among primitive people groups today, and history indicates they were virtually unknown among the oldest civilizations. The evidence indicates most ancient people consumed a diet very similar to the diet of the Bible and the original intent of our Creator.

Of course, other factors figure in our health picture as well—genetics, environmental toxins, emotional and mental characteristics, lifestyle choices, and cultural trends that affect health—but diet remains the single most influential factor in overall human health.

Tilt Some Stereotypes

When you picked up this book and looked at the title, *The Maker's Diet*, you may have classified the author—me—as a wimpy vegetarian health guru or militant vegan. If so, allow me to tilt some stereotypes for you:

1. I am in favor of eating beef, lamb, and other healthy red meats.
2. I'm a huge fan of organic, grass-fed dairy products, especially cultured dairy.
3. I believe we should intentionally spend time in direct sunlight because soaking up rays is healthy for you.
4. I'm a proponent of letting your children play in the dirt.

5.   I think we should eat more fats, especially saturated fats like those found in coconut oil, butter, and red meat.

While I readily admit that we can't go back to the old ways of our primitive ancestors, we can learn from their wisdom to overcome or avoid the modern diseases of civilization. We can make our bodies strong and more disease-resistant if we take the necessary steps to do so.

The ultimate health wisdom available to us is a diet based on health principles clearly described in the Bible, which I have called "the Maker's Diet." My health plan is remarkably well balanced and extremely healthy. Returning to the Maker's Diet as the ultimate primitive diet, based on instructions from the Creator Himself, is certain to contribute to better health for all who choose to do so.

Ambushed by Our Technology

Our technology and advances in knowledge have ambushed us because our technological and marketing skills have advanced far quicker than our digestive tracts.

We make processed foods so that they will last for years or even decades on a store shelf, adding emulsifiers like monoglycerides and diglycerides to extend shelf life, as well as preservatives with polysyllabic names that only an organic chemist can pronounce—or understand.

And don't get me started on the introduction of genetically modified crops into foods, which was in its infancy when the Maker's Diet was originally released. Using genetically modified organisms (GMOs), scientists splice together the genes of one species into another to "custom design" a selected end product. Countless forms of these bioengineered grains and fruits are offered to unsuspecting consumers in America's largest grocery stores— usually with no notice or explanation. Nearly all the major cereal makers use GMO grains.

The concept of producing pest-proof crops may sound good, but think about the ramifications. Even though incredible technological advancements in food are at our fingertips, our bodies are still genetically wired to function best on the foods favored by our ancestors.

Want to Be Healthier Than Your Neighbor?

One people group stands out among the many primitive cultures studied by anthropologists, health professionals, and nutritional historians.

This group of people carefully restricted the eating of scavengers (unclean meats like crustaceans and vultures), consumed foods rich in nutrients, and lived a lifestyle that kept them free from illnesses and plagues throughout history—as promised in Exodus 15:26. That group was the nation of Israel, the chosen people of God.

The Israelites of antiquity followed a diet established by God and were consistently healthier than all of their neighbors. Regardless of your religious preference, it's my hope that any honest student of the Scriptures will understand that the wisdom of the Bible extends far beyond the spiritual issues to encompass every area of life—including dietary, hygienic, and moral guidelines.

Peter Rothschild, M.D., Ph.D., wrote an unpublished book entitled *The Art of Health.* In a chapter called "Please Don't Eat the Wrapper," he had this to say:

> It suddenly dawned on us that God, the greatest master nutritionist of all times, has given us an all-purpose diet more than 3,000 years ago....
>
> There is abundant historic evidence that the average Israelite, up to the end of the last century [meaning 1900], lived much longer than the average Gentile. We wish to emphasize that we are referring to the Israelites up to the end of the last century, because up to those years, the overwhelming majority of Jews obeyed God's laws by and large.

However, beginning with World War I, both diet and hygiene began to slacken among the children of Israel all over the planet, until only a small fraction remains true to biblical tradition....worldwide statistics bear witness to their changing eating habits. The trend of longevity is gradually vanishing among the non-observant. It appears that God indeed knew what nourishment to recommend.

Let's go back to the beginning. In the very first chapter of the Bible, God says, "I give you every seed-bearing plant on the face of the whole earth and every tree that has fruit with seed in it. They will be yours for food" (Gen. 1:29, NIV).

This biblical provision for food, as incorporated into the Maker's Diet, provides a great amount of vitamins, minerals, protein, healthy fats, and phytochemicals, the invaluable natural substances in plants that are neither vitamins nor minerals. A wealth of nutrition awaits hurting bodies fed with liberal doses of fruits, vegetables, herbs, lentils, and properly prepared whole grains—along with the meat, fish, and dairy products introduced later by the Creator.

Apart from the de-branned, bleached, chemically stripped, and "enriched" wheat flour we use to add fat to America's "waist"-land, these biblical seed-bearing plants are rare in modern diets. That is unfortunate.

Outdated Legalism

In an odd twist of logic, many religious Americans dismiss the Jewish dietary laws as outdated legalism, invalid for the modern era. Yet they embrace the fundamental truths of the Ten Commandments as universal and timeless. So my point is this: Shouldn't we at least *consider* the Creator's dietary guidelines in the same way?

It should be noted that God gave His moral law and His dietary guidelines to the Jews at the same time. The moral guidelines preserved spiritual purity, social order, family stability, and community prosperity and were used by America's founders to establish the Constitution, building on the proven principles from the commandments God gave the Israelites thousands of years ago.

On the other hand, God's dietary guidelines to the Hebrew people preserved their physical health. His dietary guidelines were not some narrow-minded religious exercise meant to set apart certain people from their neighbors. They were given by a loving God to save His people from physical devastation long before scientific principles of hygiene, viral transmission, bacterial infection, or molecular cell physiology were understood!

Divine Dietary Revision

Many of us have heard the rationale for various "Genesis diets" championed by sincere and intelligent health experts over the years. These diets are based on Genesis 1:29, which gave Adam and Eve instructions to eat liberally from the plant foods lavishly provided in the Garden of Eden.

After Adam and Eve's exodus from the Garden of Eden, however, the proteins unique to animal foods became increasingly important to human beings who were now dependent on heavy labor, physical strength, and speed to survive. God codified approved animal protein sources in Leviticus 11 and Deuteronomy 14 in the Old Testament. I have summarized this divine dietary revision in the following chart.

SUMMARY OF THE MAKER'S DIET

The foods approved by God as recorded in Leviticus 11 and Deuteronomy 14 superseded "the Genesis Diet" found in the first chapter of the Bible. God declared, "These are the animals which you may eat among all the animals that are on the earth" (Lev. 11:2, NKJV). Abraham, Moses, Jacob, and Jesus ate biblically clean meats. Because we aren't in the Garden of Eden, we all need animal protein. The Bible is very specific on what meat can and cannot be eaten:

* The meat of animals with a cloven or split hoof that also chew the cud (Lev. 11:3) can be eaten. This includes cows, goats, sheep, oxen, deer, buffalo, and so forth.

* The meat of animals such as the camel, which chew the cud but do not have cloven or split hooves (Lev. 11:4), cannot be eaten. This biblical injunction includes, but is not limited to, horses, rats, skunks, dogs, cats, squirrels, and possums.

* The meat of swine (pigs) cannot be eaten. They have divided hooves, but they do no chew the cud. These are *unclean* animals (Lev. 11:7–8). In fact, pigs are so unclean that God warns us not to even touch the body, meat, or carcass of a pig. The Hebrew words used to describe "unclean meats" can be translated as "foul, polluted, and putrid." The same terms were used to describe "human waste" and other disgusting substances.

* On the other hand, we may eat any fish with fins and scales, but we must avoid fish or water creatures without them (Lev. 11:9–10). Those to steer clear of include smooth-skinned

species such as catfish or eel and hard-shelled crustaceans such as crab, lobster, or clams.

* We can eat birds that live primarily on insects, grubs, or grains, but we stay away from birds or fowl that eat flesh (whether caught live or carrion). They are unclean. For a complete, see Leviticus 11:13–19.

The Bible even describes edible and inedible insects in Leviticus 11:20–23, although these foods are not normally consumed in North America. Unclean "swarming things" such as lizards, moles, mice, chameleons, and crocodiles listed in verses 29–31 are also to be avoided.

The late Elmer Josephson was a pastor, missionary, and cancer survivor. In his landmark volume *God's Key to Health and Happiness,* he wrote:

> Some ask, why did the Lord make the unclean animals? Answer: they were created as scavengers. As a rule, they are meat-eating animals that clean up anything that is left dead in the fields, etc. But scavengers were never created for human consumption. The flesh of the swine is said by many authorities to be the prime cause of much of our American ill health, causing blood diseases, weakness of the stomach, liver troubles, eczema, consumption, tumors, cancer, etc.
>
> The scaleless fish and all shellfish including the oyster, clam, lobster, shrimp, etc., modern science discovers to be but lumps of devitalized and disease producing filth, because of inadequate excretion. These are the scavengers, the garbage containers of the waters and the seas.

Pork products, in particular, top the list of favorite foods for many Americans. Some don't even realize their favorite snacks or foods come from swine—like Jell-O gelatin, chicken sausages, or the All-American standard—the hot dog.

The pig did not make the Creator's list of "clean" animals for a very good reason. Clean animals that chew the cud have an alimentary canal and a secondary cud receptacle. Essentially, they have three stomachs to process and refine their clean, vegetation-based food that sustains their bodies (their flesh) in a process that takes more than twenty-four hours.

Pigs or swine, on the other hand, never limit their diet to green vegetation found in fields. They will eat anything they can find—including their own young and sick or dead pigs from the same pen.

Josephson claimed the pig's single stomach arrangement was very simple in design and function in keeping with a limited excretory organ system. "Four hours after the pig has eaten his polluted swill and other putrid, offensive matter, man may eat the same [swill] second-handed off the ribs of the pig."

Regarding scavengers of the sea, there seem to be media warnings about toxic crabs, clams, and oysters on the East Coast every spring or summer. Why? Scientists literally gauge the contaminate levels of our oceans, bays, rivers, and lakes by measuring the mercury and biological toxin levels in the flesh of crabs, clams, oysters, and lobsters.

So all this means that eating lobster, scampi, and bacon-topped cheeseburgers is problematic. Consider Dr. Rothschild's explanation of the toxic effects of what the Bible calls "unclean" foods:

> Do not consume any meat of scavenger animals comprising pork, all shellfish varieties, skin fish that are scale-less fish, scavenger birds, snakes, and most reptiles. The reason for this [biblical] prohibition is dual.
>
> The first reason is that the meat of such animals is about ten times more perishable, difficult to preserve, than that of the allowed animals. Frequently people do not realize a piece of meat is already poisonously spoiled until they perceive the toxic symptoms...[and have already] ingested it.
>
> The second reason consists in the scary fact that the...byproducts that originate from digesting such scavenger meat are highly poisonous. We're referring specifically to the so-called death enzymes, such as cadaverine, putrescine...these death enzymes are extraordinarily useful in nature. Without their assistance, no flesh would revert to dust...they are extremely useful to break down a corpse, but terribly inconvenient in a living human body.

Refined and Processed Foods

God's dietary guidelines contain no refined or processed carbohydrates and only a very small amount of healthy sweeteners. The typical American diet is just the opposite. We stray far from God's design with an array of techno-foods rich in empty calories, filled with refined carbohydrates, and woefully inadequate in nutrition.

In contrast, the totally natural Maker's Diet will satisfy you with unprocessed foods harvested directly from the Creator's bounty. Countless healing miracles occur naturally as our bodies process and use these foods with great ease.

Practice Good Hygiene as Well

Clear-cut hygiene guidelines also accompany the Maker's instructions. Generations of Jewish families have followed these instructions and enjoyed remarkable resistance to diseases and plagues, which devastated neighboring people groups with no such guidelines.

Michael D. Jacobson, D.O., a former U.S. Army flight surgeon and family practitioner, noted that in the mid-14th century, the bubonic plague wiped out one-fourth of Europe's population in just one year. The deadly contagion returned repeatedly over the next 250 years, killing nearly a fourth of London's population in 1603. At one point, England lost nearly half of its total population to this plague. Here is history's record of how the Jewish people fared in the face of such a terrible menace upon the land:

> As the plague continued its scourge, it became apparent that the Jewish people were somehow escaping its death grip. This led many to persecute them. People concluded that it was the Jews who were responsible for the plague since they were the only ones who were not dying.
>
> The truth is that, hundreds of years prior to the discovery of bacteria, the Jews were protecting themselves from the deadly *Yersinia pestis* microbe by practicing cleanliness and good hygiene….
>
> More than three thousand years before man discovered bacteria, the Creator had given detailed instructions that, if followed, would prevent the spread of such a deadly communicable disease.

In other words, the Jewish people of that day buried their solid waste and boiled water before drinking it. They also ate foods that were kosher, meaning they were not prohibited in Leviticus and Deuteronomy, and consumed kosher dairy products and did not combine meat and dairy, meaning no cheeseburgers.

Members of my Jewish family have followed kosher dietary guidelines for generations—with a few exceptions. My grandmother Rose always served her family kosher foods in the home, but she had one blind spot. "The only place we eat traife"—the Yiddish word for biblically unclean meats such as pork and shrimp—"is at a Chinese restaurant."

Grandma knew that pork and shrimp were biblically unclean foods, but she considered them acceptable to eat as long as they were not served in her home. I'm afraid that she—along with millions of others—missed the point. Even though my grandmother is no longer with us today, she would agree that her "logic" did not change the potential ill effects of those meats.

Choosing a Better Way

Some of us diligently search for the claims on prepackaged food reassuring us they are "enriched with 12 vitamins" or that they are "100 percent natural."

The unfortunate truth is that most prepackaged and fast-food products overload our bodies with adulterated fats and refined sugars such as those found in candy, baked goods, and refined grains. (That includes the ubiquitous hamburger buns and "wholesome bread" wrapped around our "low-fat" grilled chicken breasts.)

Should we give up and just eat twigs, leaves, and berries the rest of our lives? No, we don't have to be that extreme. There is a better way.

The Maker's Diet is a comprehensive lifestyle plan that will help you choose a better way to eat and to live. By way of introducing some general guidelines here, you can choose wild game instead of artificially fattened and estrogen-enhanced slabs of feedlot-raised beef. Reaching for naturally fermented raw dairy products instead of antibiotic-laced, hormone-enhanced, and pesticide-tainted pasteurized and homogenized dairy products will result in a big upgrade in your health.

I urge you to select wild fish with fins and scales instead of farm-raised varieties dosed with antibiotics. Be sure to seek out nutritious fermented or sprouted whole-grain bread (more on this tasty alternative later) instead of commercially produced white bread that tastes like sawdust and is about as nutritious. Spice up your life with naturally fermented relishes and condiments instead of sugary sauce substitutes.

Discard the Myths About Primitive People

Modern society is riddled with myths about primitive people being brutish, savage, and of low intelligence. This "caveman" mentality permeates our literature and media, but it's still the stuff of myths. We could learn a great deal from our ancestors if we lay down some of our misconceptions about nutrition.

Most of us have an image of our ancestors' primitive lifestyles that paints them as scavengers constantly on the move for something to eat. They are pictured as undernourished, animalistic, filthy, and virtually semi-human people plagued by illness and ignorance. In truth, however, many of our ancestors experienced robust health, often right up to death.

Though a high percentage of people in primitive societies died during infancy or while still young, it was largely because technological advances in modern medicine and basic knowledge about sanitation were unavailable. (Again, the Jewish people of the Bible were the significant exception because of God's sanitation guidelines given to them in Leviticus 11 and Deuteronomy 14.)

What Is a Nursing Home?

You've probably not thought about this, but your great-great-great-grandparents living at the turn of the 19th century probably could not relate to terms like *retirement* or *nursing home*. This was at a time when nearly 40 percent of the population lived and worked on a farm. Those who lived in cities didn't have cars, so they had to walk everywhere. There was so Social Security or IRA retirement accounts. You worked until you were no longer able, and then one of your children took care of you.

Most of their generation lived vigorous lifestyles filled with a lot of exercise and consumed a diet that was well suited to their bodies. This combination tended to keep them strong and healthy well into their eighties. Though some people in the past failed to live long enough to acquire cardiovascular disease or cancer (two of the major killers in the United States and Europe today), those who did live long lives rarely acquired these killer diseases.

Cardiovascular Disease Was Nonexistent

Heart disease (as well as cancer) is still rare among isolated primitive groups in the modern era who eat a more primitive, ancestral diet. One clinical study examined cardiovascular disease incidence and related risk factors among 2,300 "subsistence horticulturists"—people who survive on what they grow, gather, or harvest—on Kitava, a tropical island near Papua New Guinea in the South Pacific. The title of the study says it all: "Apparent Absence of Stroke and Ischaemic Heart Disease."

What was their secret?

Researchers determined that the modern disease symptoms of sudden cardiac death, stroke, and exertion-related chest pain were nonexistent or extremely rare in Kitavans. It seemed that the most common causes of death were infections, accidents, complications of pregnancy, and senescence (old age). All of the adults had low diastolic blood pressure (all below 90) and were very lean. (Their average weight actually decreased after age thirty.)

What did they eat most of the time? They lived on Kitava's island bounty of tubers, fruit, fish, and coconut, with very little salt and virtually no access to Western food or alcohol. Oddly enough, 80 percent of the population (both sexes) were daily smokers, supporting the concept that smoking alone is not sufficient to cause cardiovascular disease. The tobacco these native people smoked was, no doubt, grown without the use of toxic pesticides and herbicides and was smoked from a wood pipe or hand-rolled in thin paper free from chemically treated filters and glue. Thus, modern people have even found a way to make smoking even less healthy.

There was an anomaly among those surveyed—a forty-four-year-old businessman who grew up on Kitava but lived elsewhere. He had returned to visit family during the survey and agreed to participate anyway. Compared to the local Kitavan adults, this urban man had the highest diastolic blood pressure, the highest body mass index, and the highest waist-to-hip ratio.

The contrast strongly indicates that neither the Kitavans—nor any native cultures still in existence—are genetically protected from hypertension or abdominal obesity. Their good health was certainly directly linked to their healthy diet and lifestyle.

The Hidden Cost of Being Thoroughly Modern

Modern civilization has managed to infiltrate the culture of many of these once-isolated societies. Few of them today still consume the primitive, simple diets of their ancestors. American travelers are often surprised to find canned Western-style food—Spam is a huge favorite throughout the Hawaiian Islands—as well as refined sugar and white flour products consumed nearly everywhere on the planet. As you might expect, this transition from primitive diets to modern diets has brought about deadly consequences.

Explaining an Absence of Cancer

Appreciation for the virtues of a primitive diet is controversial, but it isn't new. More than a century ago, in 1913, the Nobel Prize-winning physician and missionary Albert Schweitzer visited Gabon, Africa, and had this to say:

> I was astonished to encounter no cases of cancer. I saw none among the natives two hundred miles from the coast....I cannot, of course, say positively that there was no cancer at all, but, like other frontier doctors, I can only say that if any cases existed, they must have been quite rare. This absence of cancer seemed to be due to the difference in nutrition of the natives compared to the Europeans.

Explorer and anthropologist Vilhjalmur Stefansson searched in vain for cases of cancer among the Inuit peoples—or Eskimos, as they were known then—while exploring the Arctic in the early 1900s. Meticulous diary entries of his experiences and observations appear throughout his book *Cancer: Disease of Civilization*. Stefansson said a whaling ship doctor named George B. Leavitt found only one cancer case in forty-nine years among the Eskimos of Alaska and Canada.

By the 1970s, however, breast cancer malignancy appeared frequently among the Inuit women after they began consuming a modern diet. Toxic chemicals from our modern foods and industries contributed to this condition.

Diabetes was rare among Australia's native Aborigines, but now this modern disease appears ten times more often among the Aborigines than among European arrivals. Kerin O'Dea, a professor at Monash University in Clayton, Victoria, attributes the diabetes increase to dietary changes. The flaws in our modern diet invariably produce modern diseases and a decreased quality of life.

Ironically, the Australian Aborigines used to eat great amounts of fermented sweet potatoes (a natural source of probiotics and soluble fiber that feeds the "good" bacteria of the gastrointestinal tract). These potatoes are naturally sweet, but when eaten plain or in fermented form, they seem to significantly reduce the risk of blood sugar imbalances.

Unfortunately, sweet potatoes in any form rarely make it onto our favorite foods list.

The Surprising Discoveries of Dr. Weston Price

Dr. Weston A. Price, who was born in 1870 and died in 1948, was a Harvard-trained dentist with a curious mind and a determination to find root causes. Many refer to him as the "Albert Einstein of nutrition."

I consider him to be the greatest nutritionist who ever lived. He was thrust into nutritional research after he became alarmed by the number of cavities, crooked teeth, and deformed dental arches in his young patients.

Dr. Price believed dental health was a good indicator of physical health, so he wondered if the epidemic of dental abnormalities that he was seeing in his practice were caused by nutritional deficiencies. Solid scientific evidence at the time indicated that all three symptoms Dr. Price noted in his young patients signaled physical degeneration and an increased vulnerability to diseases such as heart attacks and cancer.

Dr. Price's search for answers led him to turn from his test tubes and microscopes and launch a six-year expedition to five continents so that he could study primitive societies. He and his wife, Florence, began their travels in 1930 just as many of these societies were adopting modern diets as a result of their exposure to "outsiders." The Prices produced countless photographs and invaluable data on the dental state, dietary habits, and lifestyles of thousands of people in many primitive societies.

This gave Dr. Price the unique opportunity to compare people who had grown up with the primitive diet against those in that culture who had started consuming modern diets. (Sometimes the individuals lived in the same family or household.)

Dr. Price traveled the globe by ship and by plane in search of these isolated human groups. He studied farmers and goat shepherds in an isolated valley high in the Swiss Alps, Gaelic communities in the Outer Hebrides, the Inuit or Eskimo people of Canada and Alaska, native American Indians of North America, Melanesian and Polynesian South Sea Islanders, African tribes, Australian Aborigines, New Zealand Maori, and the Indians of South America.

Primitive Diets Produce Beautiful Teeth, Strong Bodies

Dr. Price found that primitive people consuming their traditional diets exclusively typically enjoyed beautiful straight teeth that were free of decay and strong bodies that demonstrated a remarkable resistance to disease.

He was determined to find the factors responsible for such attributes among these primitive people. He concluded that the dental caries—progressive destruction of teeth by decay—and deformed dental arches that produced crowded, crooked teeth and an unattractive appearance were merely a sign of physical degeneration. As he had originally suspected, nutritional deficiencies appeared to be the primary cause of this physical degeneration. Dr. Price reported his findings in the book that he aptly titled Nutrition and Physical Degeneration.

The Prices' astonishing collection of photographs support his finding that primitive people cut off from modern diets generally had perfectly formed teeth and jaws with very little tooth decay. There was a stark contrast between the wide faces, perfect teeth, and perfectly formed dental arches of families who lived on a primitive diet and the narrow faces, misshapen jaws, and crooked teeth of other family members who consumed modern diets!

Modern Diets Produce Physical Degeneration

Dr. Price concluded that *diet* was the only possible factor accounting for such universal good physical health among primitive people. People who ate the modern diet suffered from physical degeneration, while those on primitive diets did not. He suggested that dietary deficiencies also contributed to poor brain development and associated social disorders such as juvenile delinquency and high crime rates.

Dr. Price dared to suggest that modern humans learn from primitives—and keep in mind that he wrote this in an era when it was fashionable to disparage and sneer at primitive people groups as "uncivilized." He strongly urged a return to the primitive diet that made our ancestors so healthy and then posed this question:

> No era in the long journey of mankind reveals in the skeletal remains such a terrible degeneration of teeth and bones as this brief modern period records. Must Nature reject our vaunted culture and call back the more obedient primitives?

When Dr. Price analyzed the foods of isolated primitive peoples, he discovered that they provided at least four times the water-soluble vitamins, calcium, and other minerals and at least ten times the fat-soluble vitamins such as A, E, and D found in modern diets. The primitive diets derived these nutrients from animal foods such as butter, fatty fish, wild game, and organ meats.

Many "Primitives" Practiced Premarital Nutrition

For many years, health practitioners—as well as most people with a dose of common sense—have understood the importance of good nutrition for mothers during pregnancy. Dr. Price's research revealed that members of primitive cultures have long understood and practiced "preconception" nutritional programs for *both* prospective parents.

What Dr. Price learned during his travels was that many tribes required a period of premarital nutrition long before a young people wed. Special foods were often given to maturing boys and girls in preparation for future parenthood, as well as to pregnant and lactating women. Dr. Price found these foods to be very rich in fat-soluble vitamins A and D—nutrients found only in animal fats.

Once married, couples usually spaced out their children to permit the mother to maintain her full health and strength and to assure the safety and physical excellence of subsequent offspring. The healthy bodies, homogeneous reproduction, emotional stability, and freedom from degenerative ills enjoyed by such primitive societies contrast sharply from modern individuals existing on the impoverished foods of civilization. I'm talking about convenience

foods filled with sugar, white flour, pasteurized milk, and chemical preservatives and additives.

Here's what happened when Dr. Price compared the nutritional intake
of primitive groups with their resistance to dental caries and freedom from
degenerative processes to the diets of modernized groups who adopted
modern foods consisting largely of white flour products, sugar, white rice,
jams, canned goods, and vegetable oils. Virtually without exception, Dr. Price
discovered that when compared to modernized diets, the primitive diets provided exceptionally high levels of calcium, phosphorus, iron, magnesium,
fat-soluble vitamins (A, D, E, K), water-soluble B vitamins (folate, pantothenic
acid, thiamin, riboflavin, niacin, B6, B12), and vitamin C.

Dr. Price's keen observations were first published in 1939 in Nutrition and
Physical Degeneration. I've summarized a few observations he made from
some of the lands he visited:

* **Switzerland:** "The isolated groups dependent on locally produced natural foods have nearly complete natural immunity
  to dental caries, and the substitution of modern dietaries for
  these primitive natural foods destroys this immunity."

* **Outer Hebrides Islands (off the coast of Scotland):** "I was
  advised that in the last fifty years the average height of Scotch
  men in some parts decreased four inches, and that this had
  been coincident with the general change from high immunity
  to dental caries to a loss of immunity in a great part of this
  general district. A study of the market places revealed that a
  large part of the nutrition was shipped into the district in the
  form of refined flours, canned goods, and sugar."

* **Alaska:** "We neither saw nor heard of a case [of arthritis] in
  the isolated groups. However, at the point of contact with the
  foods of modern civilization many cases were found, including ten bedridden cripples in a series of about twenty Indian
  [Native American] homes. Some other afflictions made their
  appearance there, particularly tuberculosis, which is taking
  a very severe toll on the children who had been born at the
  center."

- **Ethiopia:** "In one of the most efficiently organized mission schools that we found in Africa, the principal asked me to help them solve a serious problem of why it is that those families that have grown up in the mission or government schools were physically not so strong as those families who had never been in contact with the mission or government schools."

The pioneering research of Dr. Price provided solid empirical evidence that the primitive peoples he studied did not suffer from obesity, heart disease, digestive problems, or cancer at the rates we do. Thanks in large part to their primitive diets, these people groups enjoyed levels of vibrant health that have virtually been lost to modern civilization.

Health Declined with a Shift to Agriculture

The scientific analysis of skeletal and dental remains of primitive societies from the past suggests that humans before the advent of modern agriculture were stronger, bigger, and healthier than those who lived after that societal change.

In general, the health of our primitive ancestors declined whenever they shifted to agriculture as their primary food supply. This was abundantly clear at a North American research site in the Illinois Valley, one of the few sites in the United States containing an intact mortuary record dating back to when pioneers first populated the area.

Researchers also uncovered a large amount of archaeological dietary evidence. This allows us to draw some solid conclusions about health and disease in the population of this region.

One site, the Dickson Mounds in Illinois, provides enough information to establish a correlation between increased primary food production and changes in the overall health level. Researchers studied data from three time periods: the Late Woodland period (950–1100 A.D.), the Mississippian Acculturated/Late Woodland period (1100–1200 A.D.), and the Middle Mississippian period (1200–1300 A.D.).

The Late Woodland component is associated with a generalized hunting and gathering economy. Compared to the appearance of these first people at the Dickson Mounds, there was a general increase of the reliance on maize or corn as the primary food crop. The number of skeletons with nonspecific skeletal infections greatly increases as the maize dependence increases.

By the Middle Mississippian period, the infection rate had more than doubled. It seems the maize-based mono-diet produced severe iron deficiency anemia in the general population. That, in turn, decreased immunity and allowed for the great increase in infection rates.

In what is now East Georgia, maize cultivation among the "First Peoples" or Native Americans occurred only after 1150 A.D. Foraging societies before that period moved with their "game" or primary meat sources or scattered far enough apart to live off the land without depleting their natural resources. Once they began to plant and harvest maize, though, they clustered closer together and lived off of their crops.

Bone Infections Increased with Agriculture-Based Diets

Although these early diets were better than our chemically enhanced foods today, they still failed to match the healthy primitive diet patterns based on hunting and foraging for foods. Before the arrival of modern agriculture, the human diet of these primitive peoples consisted mostly of meat from wild animals, fish, wild heirloom grains and seeds, vegetables, fruits, and nuts. Our bodies still crave these ancestral foods, no matter how much we think we progress technologically.

Researchers found clear evidence of increased bone infections among the new agriculturally based people groups, along with a general decrease in bone size, stature, and vigor.

But Not All Primitive Diets Are Healthy

Not all primitive diets are alike, however. Many of the cultures surrounding the Israelites back in Old Testament days were primitive, but they were riddled with diseases instigated by their diets and destructive lifestyles.

We can see this beyond our borders, too. These days, China is said to possess one of the oldest continually sustained cultures on earth, yet many in China eat foods far removed from biblical guidelines.

Back when I was writing the original *The Maker's Diet*, I spotted a headline in the *Palm Beach Post*. In bold letters, the front-page story declared, "China's Taste for Critters May Have Aided SARS," referring to the deadly flu-like epidemic that first appeared in China from late 2002 to the summer of 2003. SARS, a severe acute respiratory syndrome, killed 774 people and was the epidemic that everyone talked about before the COVID-19 pandemic hit our shores and the world with a vengeance in 2020.

At any rate, the *Palm Beach Post* article had this to say:

> The possible origin of the SARS epidemic, which made places as diverse as China, Taiwan, Hong Kong, Singapore, and Toronto no-fly zones in the past two months, has been tentatively traced to civet cats, a delicacy in omnivorous southeast China. Just as AIDS may have jumped to humans from monkeys, SARS may have found a new host in hungry human beings.

According to the reporter filing the story, civet cats were related to the mongoose. They are clearly unclean animals not meant for human consumption.

Then I couldn't help but notice this quote from the article: "The Cantonese have a saying: 'If it flies in the air and it's not an airplane, if it swims in the sea and it's not a submarine, if it has four legs and it's not a table, eat it.'"

To which I have another saying: "You are what you eat."

The Creator's Wisdom

Our Creator established our genetic and nutritional requirements long ago. He caused our ancestors to adapt to the types of foods they could gather, and there is no evidence to suggest that modern humans are any different. Despite our technological advancements, our physical bodies are still designed to consume and thrive on the same foods in the same proportions that our primitive ancestors ate thousands of years ago.

The wisdom in our physiology and biochemistry cry out for a primitive, biblical diet with plentiful amounts of healthy meat, fish, fruit, vegetables, dairy, grains, nuts, and seeds. We have departed so far from the wisdom of our forefathers that probably two-thirds of the American diet are "new foods" not designed by the Creator or eaten by our ancestors.

If we ever hope to be counted among the world's healthiest people, we must leave behind our disease-producing diets and lifestyle and return to our Creator's dietary guidelines, as incorporated in the Maker's Diet!

3

Life and Death in a Long Hollow Tube:
The Importance of the GI Tract

WHETHER YOU'RE OLD OR YOUNG, TOO MANY OF US ARE USED TO FEEL-ing crummy and being compromised in what we physically can and cannot do in life.

Americans seem to accept poor health as a normal consequence of aging, while many experience poor health while they're still young due to obesity-related diseases. If they only knew their troubles started with what they ate and put into their gut. It seems like every day researchers gather more evidence affirming the importance of the gut to overall health.

A growing cohort of health professionals believe the key to a good life—or premature death—begins in the long hollow tube called the gastrointestinal tract. Regarding the latter, 40 percent of Americans who die each year perish prematurely from preventable diseases, according to a recent study from the Centers for Disease Control and Prevention. The four leading causes of death are:

* heart disease
* cancer
* lower respiratory diseases
* stroke

Given these life-threatening diseases that afflict way too many Americans, we have neglected gastrointestinal health far too long—and haven't listened to what our guts are telling us. That's a shame, especially when you realize that according to scriptures common to the Judeo-Christian tradition, the "bowels" or the "belly" are described as the seat of the emotions.

Here's an example: in the Song of Solomon, the Shulamite lover says of her betrothed (Solomon):

> My beloved put in his hand by the hole of the door, and my **bowels** were **moved** for him.
>
> —SONG OF SOLOMON 5:4 (KJV, with emphasis added)

What modern writers would consider using bowels in romantic prose—or the word gut for that matter? They wouldn't, but maybe they should because the word gut reflects a highly accurate view of the intestinal tract. The Merriam-Webster Dictionary defines gut as:

1. the basic visceral or emotional part of a person
2. part of the alimentary canal and especially the intestine or stomach

Listening to Your Gut

Have you ever had a "gut feeling"?

Sure, you have. We all do, although some choose to ignore what their gut is telling them because they were taught in childhood to "follow reason." They believe the brain is essentially the "boss" of the body.

While it's true that the brain is the centerpiece of our mental capacity and nervous system, it's also a certain fact that there are nearly one hundred million nerve cells in the gut alone—about the same number found in the spinal cord!

One-half of your nerve cells are located in the gut, so it's logical that your capacity for feeling and emotional expression can come from the gut, followed to a lesser extent by your brain. By the time you add together the number of nerve cells in the esophagus, stomach, and small and large intestines, there are more nerve cells in the overall digestive system than anywhere else in the peripheral nervous system.

When people say the brain determines whether you are happy or sad, they have their facts skewed. The gut is more responsible than you can ever imagine for mental well-being and how you feel.

Actually, You Have Two Brains

Award-winning science writer Sandra Blakeslee specializes in "cognitive neuroscience." She captured the link between our gut and the brain perfectly in this quote from one of her numerous *New York Times* articles:

> Have you ever wondered why people get butterflies in the stomach before going on stage? Or why an impending job interview can cause an attack of intestinal cramps? And why antidepressants targeted for the brain cause nausea or abdominal upset in millions of people who take such drugs?
>
> The reason for these common experiences is because each of us literally has two brains—the familiar one encased in our skulls and a lesser-known but vitally important one found in the human gut. Like Siamese twins, the two brains are interconnected; when one gets upset, the other does, too.

This "second brain" in the gut is called the enteric nervous system (ENS)—enteric being a Greek term for "intestine." This intestinal nervous system consists of neurons, neurotransmitters, and messenger proteins embedded in the layers or coverings of tissues that line the esophagus, stomach, small intestine, and colon.

The enteric nervous system possesses a complex neural circuitry, and this "second brain" in your gut acts independently from the first brain in your body. Literally, the second brain learns from experiences, remembers past actions and events, and produces an entire range of "gut feelings" that influences your actions.

Has anyone ever advised you to "follow your gut" or "go by instinct"? They may not have known it at the time, but they were telling you to listen to your second brain.

Two Nervous Systems Form During Fetal Development

Early in our embryogenesis, a collection of tissue called the "neural crest" appears and divides during fetal development. One part turns into the central nervous system, and the other migrates to become the enteric nervous system. Both "thinking machines" form simultaneously and independently of one another until a later stage of development.

Then the two nervous systems link through a neural cable called the vagus nerve, the longest of all cranial nerves. The name comes from a Latin root meaning "wandering," which makes sense because the vagus nerve "wanders" from the brain stem through organs in the neck and thorax before finally terminating in the abdomen. This is your vital brain-gut connection.

I've coined the term gastro-neuro-immunology to describe the profound influence and importance of this link between our two brains and its effect on human immune function.

Never Underestimate Your Second Brain

The mass of gray matter between your ears is immensely important to your well-being, but after what I've just described about your "second gut," you should never discount the vital importance of the gut.

Dr. Michael Gershon, chairman of the department of anatomy and cell biology at Columbia University in New York City, has devoted his career to understanding the human bowel. He described the body's second nervous system in his landmark book *The Second Brain* in this fashion:

> The brain is not the only place in the body that's full of neurotransmitters. A hundred million neurotransmitters line the length of the gut, approximately the same number that is found in the brain... The brain in the bowel has got to work right or no one will have the luxury to think at all.

There's a lot of work going on in the gut, which started getting medicine's attention at the end of the 19th century. Around 1899, two English physiologists at University College in London first discovered and described the interaction of hormones at the command of neural cells (ganglion) in the digestive tract. When William M. Bayliss and Ernest H. Starling anesthetized dogs in 1902, they applied pressure to the interior cavity of the intestine. The pressure caused contraction and relaxation followed by a propulsive wave. This propulsive wave or peristaltic reflex became known as the "law of the intestine" and describes the way the intestine propels food through the digestive tract.

Follow-up experimental studies by Drs. Bayliss and Starling demonstrated that "the law of the intestine" operated and digestion continued even when all nerves connecting the bowel to the brain and spinal cord were severed. This convinced the scientists that the enteric nervous system (ENS) was independent from the central nervous system.

A German scientist named Paul Trendelenburg confirmed the work of Bayliss and Starling eighteen years later, but the scientific community quickly refocused its interest on one of the more exciting discoveries of the day: chemical neurotransmitters such as epinephrine and acetylcholine.

Scientists Forgot the Second Brain for a While

After a political conflict within the scientific community, disgruntled scientists at the Physiological Society arbitrarily reclassified the enteric nerves as simply part of the "parasympathetic nervous system" and essentially wrote off the discovery of the "second brain" for more than a half-century.

Interest in the ENS revived between 1965 and 1967 when Dr. Michael Gershon proposed the existence of a third neurotransmitter—serotonin (5-hydroxytryptamine, 5-HT)—that was both produced in and targeted to the enteric nervous system. Dr. Gershon's proposition was confirmed, and we now know that this neurotransmitter is also found in the central nervous system.

You've probably heard of serotonin, a chemical created by the body and commonly regarded as being a chemical that makes you feel good. Serotonin is also an ingredient in over-the-counter sleep aids and is crucial for emotional health and balance. During its work as a neurotransmitter, serotonin directly affects the well-being and function of your digestive system.

We are still discovering ways the enteric nervous system mirrors the central nervous system, but one thing is clear: nearly every substance that helps run and control the brain has turned up in the gut. Major neurotransmitters associated with the brain—like serotonin, dopamine, glutamate, norepinephrine, and nitric oxide—are found in plentiful amounts in the gut as well.

The Gut Manufactures Opiates and Mood-Controllers

About twenty-four small brain proteins called neuropeptides also appear in relatively high amounts in the gut, as well as major cells of the immune system. Researchers have even found plentiful amounts of enkephalins—a class of natural opiates in the body—in the gut. The digestive system is also a rich source of benzodiazepines, which are psychoactive chemicals included in such popular mood-controlling drugs like Valium and Xanax.

Karl Lashley, whom many consider the founder of neuropsychology, said way back in 1951, "I am coming more and more to the conviction that the rudiments of every human behavioral mechanism will be found represented even in primitive activities of the nervous system."

Even back then, Lashley was on to something. This link between the brain and the gut is helping researchers understand why people act and feel the way they do.

The Importance of Sleep

Sleep disturbances set up vicious cycles of pain, fatigue, and emotional distress that make sleep even more unlikely. Things don't improve much during waking hours either for people who do not sleep well. Inadequate sleep increases sensitivity to bowel, skin, and muscle stimuli, thus leading to more pain and distress. I know from personal experience that when I don't get sufficient sleep, my digestion suffers as a result.

The brain and gut are much alike; both have natural ninety-minute cycles. The slow wave sleep of the brain is interrupted by periods of "rapid eye movement," or REM sleep, in which dreams occur. Patients with bowel problems tend to have abnormal REM sleep, and poor sleep has been reported by many patients with irritable bowel syndrome (IBS) and non-ulcer dyspepsia, otherwise known as "sour stomach."

Doctors often treat abnormal REM sleep with mild antidepressants, which may also be effective in treating IBS and non-ulcer dyspepsia, but some stronger antidepressants make digestive problems worse. Once again this points to a link between sleeping problems and stomach problems.

So, do the two brains influence each other? Answer: probably.

Sleep may very well be the single most important ingredient for digestive health, but it's also important to get enough sleep at the right time. Some researchers believe that every minute you sleep before midnight is the equivalent of four minutes of sleep after midnight, which is why I'm diligent about getting to bed by 10 p.m. Restful sleep will do wonders for your digestion and overall health.

Things Go Wrong When Serotonin Is Robbed from the Gut

Many prescription drugs that affect the brain also affect the gut. Some individuals who take Prozac or similar antidepressants may experience gastrointestinal problems such as nausea, diarrhea, and constipation. What happens is that these drugs divert serotonin from the body to the brain. Unfortunately, this leaves less serotonin for the cells of the gastrointestinal tract and leaves the door open to an upset stomach.

Normally, the gut produces more serotonin than any other part of the body. This is important because serotonin is linked with initiation of peristalsis, or the rhythmic movement of food through the digestive tract. When that supply of serotonin is reduced or stopped altogether, everything related to food digestion goes haywire. Some doctors prescribe small doses of Prozac to treat chronic constipation, but if a little Prozac cures constipation, a lot of Prozac causes it!

Opiates also have a powerful effect on the digestive tract because the gut has opiate receptors much like the brain. Dr. Michael Loes, a pain management specialist and author of The Healing Response, wrote, "Not surprisingly, drugs like morphine and heroin that are thought to act on the central nervous system also attach to the gut's opiate receptors, producing constipation. Both brains can be addicted to opiates."

Many Alzheimer's and Parkinson's disease patients suffer from constipation because these conditions impact the "second brain" in the gut as well as the "first brain" and central nervous system.

Anxious? Follow Your Gut Feeling

Fortunately, the Creator equipped the human gut with its own ways of coping with pain and stress. As I mentioned, the gut produces benzodiazepines, the same pain-alleviating chemicals found in anti-anxiety drugs such as Valium. It seems the gut is equipped to be your body's anxiety and pain reliever!

If you overeat because you feel anxious, your body may try to use the extra food to produce more benzodiazepines. We are not sure whether the gut synthesizes benzodiazepine from chemicals in our foods, from bacterial actions, or from both. What we do know is that extreme pain appears to put the gut into overdrive in order to send benzodiazepine directly to the brain for immediate pain management.

Evidently, if you take care of your gut, it will take care of you.

Problems Ahead

A common complaint in the examination rooms of family physicians around the country is this: "Doc, there's something wrong with my stomach."

Or my gut. Or the way I go to the bathroom—or can't go.

Digestive complaints, including everything from hemorrhoids to duodenal ulcers to chronic constipation, result in more time lost at work, school, and play than any other health-related problem.

Interestingly enough, according to epidemiological research done by Dr. Weston A. Price, Dr. Albert Schweitzer, and other pioneering doctors, many of these digestive problems were rare or nonexistent a century ago. What did our ancestors know or do that we do not?

For one thing, they ate a diet similar to the Maker's Diet and maintained physically vigorous lifestyles. We, on the other hand, tend to eat whatever we want at the drive-thru window or from take-out and are tethered to our computers, tablets, and smartphones, meaning we don't move around very much. This type of lifestyle costs us dearly.

When we continually eat wrong foods that are rarely digested properly, these byproducts of incomplete digestion clog the gut with accumulated debris and become a perfect breeding ground for dangerous forms of bacteria and other microorganisms.

So, if you're nodding your head and looking to make a lifestyle change by adopting the Maker's Diet, I have some good news for you. There are some very positive things you can do to reverse any damage that has already been done. I know because after Crohn's disease all but decimated my body's digestive system, intestinal cleansing or detoxification was one of the keys to overcoming my illness.

Even though I visited the bathroom nearly ten thousand times over the two years I was sick—that's an average of thirteen times a day for those of you keeping score at home—I still needed to be cleansed. I went through a natural detoxification process by introducing beneficial microorganisms into my body that helped me regain the natural balance of microflora in my gut.

A Look at Self-Poisoning

A couple of years before I wrote *The Maker's Diet*, I appeared on a series of television programs devoted to health issues. A viewer watched one of my interviews and felt compelled to send me a medical textbook written in in 1896 that examined the problems associated with autointoxication, which is defined as self-poisoning from the body's absorption of toxins and waste products.

Surprisingly, autointoxication was a recognized cause of disease in the late 1900s and early 20th century. Dr. H.H. Boeker, who studied the digestive tract, stated in 1928, "It is now universally conceded that autointoxication is the underlying cause of an exceptionally large group of symptom complexes."

Today's research seems to support these earlier conclusions about intestinal toxemia, yet many modern medical practitioners and researchers still dismiss intestinal toxemia as an old and outdated concept.

We need to get back to the basics. The gut goes from your mouth all the way to the "other end." It is fully self-contained and yet intricately dependent and interlinked with every other major system of your body. It's becoming clearer that anything you come into contact with, such as swimming and showering in chlorinated water, swallowing fluoride toothpaste, wearing synthetic clothing, or even cleaning house with powerful chemicals, may indirectly or directly affect your gut and therefore your health.

In fact, virtually every state of health is affected by the GI tract. Even if you break a bone or undergo a surgical procedure, the time required to heal is directly affected by how well your gut can process body-building nutrients and detoxify toxins!

I don't care if you're the most intelligent person in the world, but if you fail to fuel your body properly, your brilliant intellect may be dimmed or extinguished through poor nutrition and poor lifestyle decisions.

Digestion: The Law of the Gut

We can accurately say that the digestive process is ruled by the "law of the gut." Simply defined, digestion is:

- a carefully executed decomposition process
- carried out by an independent enteric nervous system
- supported by an intricate array of interactive enzymes

The food you eat yields only a small proportion of substances usable by your body. The rest is eliminated as two fundamental kinds of waste: metabolic waste and digestive waste.

Metabolic waste represents the cellular household waste and the breakdown of dead, discarded cells that are constantly being replaced in the body. Most metabolic waste is eliminated through the kidneys via your urine. (Less than 4 percent exits the body through the bowels.)

Digestive waste comprises all the broken-down matter from the digestion process that is not absorbed. If these waste products are not regularly eliminated via a bowel movement, they can poison the body and blood. Unchecked, this autointoxication may lead to disease and even death.

Throughout history, people from virtually every ethnic group or nationality have in their folklore an instinctive understanding about the importance of regular elimination in the form of daily, comfortable bowel movements. My Jewish grandmother told me her mother often used an old Yiddish expression to describe her day-to-day digestive health. If someone asked her, "Mama, are you hungry?" she would reply, "No, dis bachala teet vay." (I've spelled the phrase phonetically.)

The translation: "No, my stomach isn't clean."

Her mother—my great-grandmother—usually refused to eat until she had a bowel movement that day because she had learned through experience how important it was to detoxify the body and cleanse the colon. Most modern Americans don't follow her benchmark. They'll wake up and have a big bowl of sugar-crusted cereal and a sesame bagel with a schmear of cream cheese to go with their morning coffee and give nary a thought about the last time they had a bowel movement. Then it's off to the office, constipated and backed up like nobody's business. When they feel bloated and get too far behind, they take a toxic, chemical-based laxative or schedule a visit to the doctor's office, where the merry-go-round continues.

Unfortunately, disease may visit those who feast and live foolishly. It concerns me that adults and children have unhealthy standards of digestion and elimination. Some elementary school children are told in health classes that two bowel movements per week should be considered normal!

Dr. H.H. Boeker believed nearly a hundred years ago that over 90 percent of diseases are caused or complicated by toxins created in the intestinal tract by unhealthy foods that are not properly eliminated. I wonder where he'd put that number today. Ninety-nine percent?

What everyone agrees on is that autointoxication occurs when—due to poor elimination—certain toxins escape from the bowel into the blood stream and poison the body, causing a silent form of self-poisoning.

Two Keys to Optimal Health

Guidelines for optimal health and nutrition can be reduced to two vital keys:

1. Optimize the nutrition entering your body.
2. Reduce the toxins in your body.

Virtually every disease can be related to those two guidelines in some way—and it all starts in the small and large intestines.

Caring for Your Colon

The colon is the number one repository for oxidative stress in the body. Perhaps you've heard a great deal in the media about antioxidants and the danger of free radicals, but very few realize that most of the free radicals or oxidative damage is generated in the colon during the final stages of the digestion process. This explains why it's good to eliminate waste *daily* rather than have it languish for days in the digestive tract, generating potentially harmful toxins all the while.

Necessary Enzymes

Our ancestors enjoyed exceptional health partly because they regularly consumed foods rich in enzymes and probiotics—vital nutrients that remain a mystery to most Americans.

Enzymes play a key role in a healthy gut by helping your digestive system break down proteins, fats, sugars, starches, and other carbohydrates. Your body requires a steady supply of enzymes to digest food properly and maintain health. Thousands of different enzymes exist in nature, but they may be divided into two basic categories.

The first category, **lytic enzymes**, is designed and programmed to break down only specified substances. For example, proteolytic enzymes break down proteins only, without affecting fats or sugars.

The second category of enzymes, **synthetic enzymes**, focuses exclusively on the process of synthesis in the body and is uniquely equipped to help create new substances or structures such as molecules and tissues.

The human body produces most of the enzymes it needs, but certain key enzymes such as cellulase—an enzyme that breaks down the fiber contained in plant foods—must be obtained from raw vegetables and fruits that enter the digestive system. These enzymes and the complex processes of the digestive tract are vitally related to good health.

If you fail to eat the proper foods, however, or if you abuse your body with poor dietary choices, consume processed foods with tons of preservatives, or pursue a grab-and-go lifestyle at convenience stores, you could lose more than your youthful appearance. Enzyme deficiency may also impair your immune function, resulting in illness or disease. High-speed, high-volume lifestyles and toxic eating habits deprive you of the enzymes you desperately need. Even worse, eating the wrong foods deteriorates the organs that produce many of the body's most crucial enzymes.

This progressive, overall depletion of enzymes leads to a no-win situation in which you can neither digest the food you eat nor synthesize the materials you need for cell repair and maintenance. Even a partial enzyme deficiency may lead to the onset of disease.

If your enzyme deficiencies grow worse, it gets harder and harder for the body to digest proteins, fats, sugars, starches, and other carbohydrates. The resulting poor digestion can open the door to a great variety of health problems.

Enter the Lymphatic System

The lymphatic system is your body's front line of defense against infection and disease. Its primary job is to defend your body from foreign invasion by disease-causing agents such as viruses, bacteria, or fungi.

The lymph system contains a network of vessels that help circulate and filter body fluids. Lymph nodes or glands dot the network of lymphatic vessels and provide meeting grounds for the immune system cells that defend against invaders. They also produce lymph, a pale fluid resembling blood plasma that contains white blood cells. (Lymph is a Greek term meaning "a pure, clear stream.")

The lymphatic fluids bathe the tissues of the body and are collected by the lymphatic vessels and discharged into the blood stream. Serious problems arise when lymph glands are blocked and this vital service to the body's cells is eliminated. Lymphatic congestion is considered one of the foremost trigger factors for a great variety of serious diseases.

Dealing with Your GALT

Sixty to 80 percent of the lymphatic system is contained in your small intestine. Called the gut-associated lymphoid tissue (GALT), it is almost synonymous with the term *immune system*. The gigantic task of your GALT is to discriminate between nutritious components and possible antigens passing through your bowel.

Isn't it incredible how God created our bodies?

Because antigens signal the presence of something that threatens the healthy cells and systems of the body, your GALT alerts the immune system to respond appropriately. When your GALT fails to function properly, however, your immune health is compromised. Dangerous toxins may escape from the colon into your bloodstream. Numerous illnesses could be released to attack virtually any tissue or organ—even your entire body.

That is why lymphomas (cancer of the lymphatic system) spread so rapidly. The lymphatic system literally goes throughout the length of your body, which is why this form of cancer is so dangerous.

Positioned Through the Body

While your GALT is the most important of all of the lymphatic systems, the lymphoid organs, or organs of the immune system, are positioned throughout the body. They include the spleen, located at the upper left of the abdomen, which is also a staging ground where immune system cells confront foreign microbes.

Pockets of lymphoid tissue appear in many other locations throughout the body such as in the bone marrow, thymus, tonsils, adenoids, Peyer's patches, and the appendix. This brief description of your body's defense system can help you understand how important it is for you to care for your colon. You do that by providing proper nutrition for your body and avoiding processed and devitalized foods, antibiotics, caffeine, alcohol, chlorine, and other toxins.

Maintaining a healthy gut, a free-flowing lymph system, and a healthy immune function happens when you include plenty of natural foods from the Maker's Diet, which are rich in enzymes, along with probiotics and a lifestyle that includes movement and exercise.

As you may know, your health is vitally connected to a vast universe of microscopic organisms that thrive in and on every living thing. A wide array of antibiotics has been unleashed to kill and destroy virtually all microorganisms.

In coming chapters, you're going to learn more regarding the critical need to avoid this "micro-mayhem." You see, many of these tiny microorganisms—the "good bacteria"—may be both the smallest and best friends you'll ever have.

≈

4

Hygiene: The Double-Edged Sword

A**N OBSCURE RACE OF PEOPLE ATTEMPTING TO CROSS THE SINAI**
Peninsula about 3,500 years ago received a highly advanced system of
disease prevention and medical hygiene.

Consider these instructions from the Lord set forth in Deuteronomy:

> Also, you shall have a place outside the camp, where you may go out;
> and you shall have an implement among your equipment, and when
> you sit outside, you shall dig with it and cover your refuse.
> —DEUTERONOMY 23:12-13 (NKJV)

That's the New King James Version, which is a more formal translation.
Here's how The Message translated the same passage of Scripture:

> Mark an area outside the camp where you can go to relieve yourselves.
> Along with your weapons have a stick with you. After you relieve
> yourself, dig a hole with the stick and cover your excrement.

Get the picture? The Hebrews were directed by God to use a wooden stick
as a shovel and bury their business.

In ancient times, this was a revolutionary development. People weren't
very sanitary in those days, but that's because there were no sewers, no toilets,
and no indoor plumbing. With people using chamber pots or open latrines
behind their stone homes, no wonder deadly diseases swept through civilizations during ancient times and into the Middle Ages, when the bubonic plague
wiped out nearly half of Europe.

The Hebrews in Moses' time were different. They followed God's instructions and escaped the communicable diseases and social ills that plagued their Gentile neighbors, as they were promised:

> If you diligently heed the voice of the Lord your God...I will put none
> of these diseases on you which I have brought on the Egyptians. I am
> the Lord who heals you.
>
> —EXODUS 15:26

Remember that the Hebrews refraining from eating certain "unclean" foods and practicing good hygiene wasn't the prevailing wisdom of the times. Moses, as a prince of Egypt, was certainly aware of Egyptian prescriptions for staying healthy or avoiding epidemics, but he did not embrace Egypt's "two vulture feathers" and the promise from a god named "Flame-in-his-face" to save them "from every sickness." History records that the Egyptians treated pinkeye with "the urine of a faithful wife" and favored other treatments such as the "blood of a worm" and a healthy plaster of the latest manure concoction! Armed with God's instructions, Moses made sure those types of "treatments" didn't fly in the Hebrew camp.

Forensic examinations of mummified Egyptians indicate the upper-class Egyptians didn't receive much benefit from the best that Egyptian physicians had to offer. They suffered from many of the same diseases that afflict us today because they also had a taste for unhealthy foods and a blatant disregard for hygiene.

The Practice of Advanced Hygiene

In contrast, the Israelites followed hygienic practices like burying their waste according to the divine instructions given to Moses. Result: they enjoyed an extraordinary resistance to sickness and disease. I'm happy to report that God's hygiene system is remarkably up to date. In fact, modern hospitals everywhere follow nearly every one of the original guidelines God laid out in the Bible.

Let me describe some of those. For example, the biblical hygiene regimen recorded in Numbers 19:11-22 required strict separation of the corpses of the dead from the living. When a person died, those present and anyone who prepared the body for burial (mandated before sundown) were considered unclean for seven days.

Those individuals were to wash their hands, clothing, and utensils with running water, extensive scrubbing, and a mild astringent. The water was treated with ashes—a key component of soap for millennia—and administered with hyssop, which contained the antiseptic thymol (which also happens to be the active ingredient in Listerine mouthwash). In addition, this biblical hygiene system required that hands be washed before meals and at other key times to ensure cleanliness.

The Bible also prescribed specific techniques for purifying clothing and key instruments or utensils, childbirth procedures, sexual hygiene, feminine hygienic guidelines (for the menses), and more.

Leviticus 13 provides detailed instructions for those with leprosy, with strict guidelines for the purification of fabrics contaminated by the disease. Scripture also called for the quarantine of people with any highly infectious disease, the most highly effective way to combat a contagion as we were reminded during the COVID-19 pandemic.

The Purpose of Advanced Hygiene

The reason I'm making big deal about proper hygiene is because cleanliness inside and out is as essential as diet and exercise to optimum health. You can significantly reduce infections, allergy attacks, and other negative health conditions by cleansing your body of toxins, pollutants, allergens, and disease-causing germs.

The direct relationship between good health and good hygiene has long been established. In fact, the first cure for cancer was based in proper hygiene. In the eighteenth century, London's chimney sweeps had an extraordinarily high rate of scrotal cancer until it was learned that those who regularly washed away the carcinogenic soot on their skin did not contract the disease.

Pioneering Modern Hygiene

One hundred years later, in the 1850s, hundreds of thousands of European women were dying of childbirth, until a Viennese obstetrician named Dr. Ignaz Semmelweis inadvertently rediscovered biblical hygiene. His medical students routinely dissected cadavers barehanded in one room and then walked into the maternity ward to perform pelvic examinations or help deliver babies—without washing their hands! Death rates for mothers in childbirth often approached the 50 percent mark.

Dr. Semmelweis was puzzled why this was happening, because expecting mothers who gave birth in their homes with midwives in attendance died in far lower numbers, something like 2 percent. In his search for answers, he decided to ask every doctor and medical student to wash their hands before entering the maternity ward.

Maybe washing up will save lives, he thought. Germs hadn't been discovered yet, but Dr. Semmelweis had an inkling that something on the hands of doctors who shuttled back and forth from the cadaver room to the delivery ward was infecting moms and their newborns.

When the doctors started giving their hands a thorough washing, the death rate for women giving birth dropped by 90 percent! Instead of being hailed by his colleagues, however, Dr. Semmelweis was ridiculed by those who felt his theory was so much…hogwash. It took another twenty or thirty years for attitudes to change—and for more medical discoveries to back him up—until Dr. Semmelweis was proven right.

Still, it was an uphill battle for a long time. It's estimated that even as late as World War II, poor hygiene caused three times more deaths than battlefield wounds.

Germs Don't Fly—They Hitchhike

We have come a long way since the days when doctors moved from one bloody or diseased patient to the next without washing their hands and changing into clean scrubs. We now know that the body's immune system is an autonomic or "automatic" function. The body reacts automatically when it senses an invasion by the disease-causing bacteria, fungi, viruses, and allergens that surround us in our homes, job sites, or backyards. Normally, the human immune system effectively fights off these diseases, but it easily becomes overloaded in today's toxic world.

To make matters worse, our trans-global travel rapidly can transport new diseases around the world in a day. Please understand that germs and microbes don't fly to the next country—they hitchhike on the hands and skin of those traveling to get there. Germs generally travel via hand-to-hand contact or hand-to-surface-to-hand transfer.

Think about it: your hands come into contact with the chief agents of infection on hundreds of surfaces daily, including other hands—and whatever they have touched. The reason for this is because more than 90 percent of the germs on your hands reside under the fingernails. The same is true for allergens and environmental contaminants.

Unfortunately, it's difficult to reach this area with normal handwashing techniques. Because they linger, these germs easily enter the body through the nasal passageways or the tear ducts of the eyes when we touch them, which occurs at least twenty times a day. Typically, your fingertips come in contact with your eyes and nose more than 12,500 times each year. Each time that happens, there is the potential of autoinoculating yourself with germs, allergens, environmental toxins, and viruses.

Autoinoculation of the eyes and nose from contaminated fingertips is particularly dangerous because the eyes and nose provide a direct pathway to the upper respiratory tract. (Some diseases enter the body through the mouth, but fluids in the mouth and stomach combat pathogens very effectively.) Upper respiratory problems, including sinus problems, account for eight of every ten visits to doctors' offices. The average adult battles two to four colds per year (six to eight colds annually for children), and nearly one person in three has allergies.

As with most instinctive human behavior, autoinoculation also serves an important positive purpose. When a baby boy first touches his fingertips to his eyes and nose, he introduces his immune system to the outside world, triggering the production of key antibodies to protect his body from infection and to preserve health. This natural process continues throughout life, keeping the immune system "attuned" to changes in the outside world.

Reducing Stress on Your Immune System

The good news is that the potentially deadly autoinoculation process is entirely avoidable. An advanced hygiene system can help you remove the overload of germs from the immune system.

The Maker's Diet program of advanced hygiene represents an advancement in how we wash up and could be the most key development since the bar of soap was invented about 175 years ago. Following this program allows the body to defend and protect itself against invasion from diseases more effectively by addressing the proper cleansing of the areas under the finger-nails and the membranes around the eyes and nose. These staging areas for germs are virtually neglected by today's popular hygiene methods.

The Maker's Diet advanced hygiene protocol preserves the balance between the proper function of autoinoculation in building the body's natural defense capabilities and its negative role in promoting infection by mass contamina-tion through the eyes and nose. Careful cleaning under the fingernails and the membranes around the eyes and nose through advanced hygiene tech-niques reduces stress on the immune system and helps reduce the occurrence of infectious disease and allergies. Once the overload is removed from the immune system, you can devote energy to eliminating other infections that are present in the body, such as lingering bronchitis or sinusitis.

I have personally been using this simple hygiene program faithfully for years, and following this system has kept me virtually free from all respira-tory illness and sinus infections. There have been times in my life when I've been on a plane every few days for weeks at a time, as well as long interna-tional flights to Europe, South Africa, Australia, and Singapore. Whether I'm on the road or home with my family, it's comforting to know that I am provid-ing myself a daily measure of protection.

Deterring Allergies

Advanced hygiene techniques thoroughly cleanse or wash away contaminants, but they do not sterilize the fingernail beds and body membranes around the eyes and nasal passages. Sterilization using antimicrobial substances does more harm than good because this process prevents the immune system from adapting to the outside environment. This is especially important where aller-gies are concerned.

More than 60 million Americans—one in every five—suffer from allergies or have an asthma infection, according to the Asthma and Allergy Foundation of America. Their suffering continues even though many have visited aller-gists, taken tests, tried shots, and ingested recommended drugs. Allergies are caused by mistaken immune system responses to harmless substances such as pollen, cat hair, or dust mites. These responses produce defensive immune symptoms such as runny noses and watering eyes.

The allergy industry treats allergies through the exclusive use of drugs that either desensitize the immune system toward potential allergens or suppress its natural response system altogether. Most of these drugs have multiple side effects and are only marginally effective. While we can't ignore the suffering, we can take a simpler, commonsense approach to the problem.

The concepts of the Maker's Diet advanced hygiene offer better cleansing techniques that will keep most of the offending substances away from your body and may even avoid triggering an immune system response altogether.

I'm astounded that this simple approach for keeping allergens away from the body is not more prevalent in our culture. I believe the failure of traditional pharmaceutical allergy treatments—the downing of pills, taking in sprays, and accepting injected drugs—to genuinely relieve allergy symptoms has triggered a strong interest in alternative methods of treatment.

If you or your family suffers from frequent colds and flu, nagging allergies, upper respiratory problems, weakened immunity, or other chronic health problems, I urge you to try the Maker's Diet method of advanced hygiene, which is described in *The Maker's Diet* 40-Day Health Experience.

The Rest of the Microbe Story

The common approach to hygiene has classified all germs (or microbes) as "bad." Actually, the Creator designed our bodies to make the maximum use of naturally occurring substances in our environment—including microbes or "germs."

Every day scientists fan out around the globe with spoons and sandwich bags in hand looking for new sources of soil microorganisms in bat caves, jungle clearings, peat bogs, hot springs, and even Egyptian mummies. Each exotic locale may yield a completely new discovery of germs—as well as a gold mine of potential pharmaceutical profits. Some leading government officials and scientists in the United States suspect that organisms in our soil may yield powerful new treatments for AIDS, cancer, and other deadly diseases. Even the National Cancer Institute is funding research on soil organisms.

We have just begun to harvest the vast resources of biological "bugs," and the search for new "super antibiotics" has never been more intense. Yet, the pool of known antibiotic formulas is growing less and less effective in the face of ever-mutating "super bugs" and infectious diseases, especially since the original Maker's Diet was released more than a decade ago. Consider these alarm bells sounded by the folks at Consumer Reports in recent years:

> The drugs we have relied on for seventy years to fight bacterial infection—everything from infected cuts to potentially deadly pneumonia—are becoming powerless. Why? Because antibiotics are often misused by doctors, patients and even people raising animals for meat. And that misuse, which includes prescribing or using those drugs incorrectly, breeds "super bugs"—dangerous, antibiotic-resistant bacteria that can't be easily controlled.

That's why the race is on and fueling so much scientific excitement about dirt. Each new dig could be the source of newly discovered microbes, different from any that have been used to date to create antibiotics. Many current antibiotics come from microbes in the soil, including streptomycin, the first treatment for tuberculosis, and vancomycin, currently the drug of last resort for the toughest infections.

You'd think that sooner or later—and it looks like sooner—scientists would run out of new places to unearth and study, but treasure hunters are still dist covering valuable microbes:

- An employee of Sandoz Pharmaceutical took a vacation in Norway and gathered a soil sample containing a mold that later led to the development of cyclosporine, the celebrated anti-rejection drug used in transplants.
- A scientist discovered microbes that can turn starch into sugar in the soil of an Indonesian temple.
- A researcher in Japan picked up a clump of soil from a golf course that produced a drug now used to cure parasitic infections plaguing livestock.

Have You Had Your Packet of 10,000 Species Yet?

Does this dusty trail on the subject of dirt seem boring to you? It doesn't have to be. Did you know that one gram of soil—enough to fill a little packet of sugar—can contain as many as 10,000 species of microbes unknown to science, according to Jo Handelsman, a professor of plant pathology at the University of Wisconsin?

Business Week notes, "Now, for the first time, [Handelsman] and her colleagues...are learning to extract the DNA of these mysterious creatures and clone it. They are finding that the microbes differ so profoundly from known bacteria that they could represent entirely new kingdoms of life—as different from other bacteria as animals are from plants. That means that the proteins produced by these creatures could have properties unlike any other known substances." Handelsman said that several new antibiotics have been identified from such soil microbes.

It Takes a Healthy "Community" to Keep Us Healthy

The same article explains the working principles of soil microbes (also called soil-based organisms, or SBOs) that helped turn around my personal health problems, and it gives understanding of why anyone with Crohn's or any other disease may well benefit from them:

> Even human intestines—an environment most people consider pretty familiar—are home to perhaps 10,000 kinds of microbes... Indeed, one of the surprises in the decoding of the human genome was that it contains more than 200 genes that come from bacteria. Microbes not only keep us alive; in some small part, we are made of them.
>
> [Researchers are] now looking at how these largely unknown microbes might play a role in Crohn's disease, an inflammation of the small intestine. [They have] found that the makeup of the mixed "community" of microbes in the intestines changes in people with the disease. A similar thing might happen with tuberculosis...leading [researchers] to wonder whether some diseases might be caused not by a single dangerous microbe, but by a change in the microbial community— an ecological imbalance inside the human body.

Countless numbers of microorganisms live in the soil, in and on plants, and in the human gut. Inside and out we are one with the earth—or should be. What depth of incomprehensible wisdom lies in the biblical statement in Genesis 2:7: "And the Lord God formed man of the dust of the [earth], and breathed into his nostrils the breath of life; and man became a living being."

Do Everyone a Favor: Come Home "Dirty"

Through the centuries, our society has migrated from living with too little hygiene—meaning being ignorant of the deadly potential of germs—to an environment that is too clean.

Twenty-five years ago, Dr. David Strachan, a respected epidemiologist at Britain's London School of Hygiene and Tropical Medicine, launched a tidal wave of debate about human immunology development and disease control by saying, "We need dirt."

Dr. Strachan proposed that society's growing separation from dirt and germs may well be the cause of weaker immune systems resulting in the growing incidence of a wide range of maladies. The British researcher advanced the "over-cleanliness theory" after noticing that children belonging to large families were much less likely to develop asthma, hay fever, or eczema.

Why was that? Dr. Strachan theorized that older children coming home dirty with all sorts of resident soil microorganisms were actually protecting their younger brothers and sisters by exposing their immune systems to microbes and causing them to build antibodies. Turns out he was on to something.

Near-epidemic waves of diseases all but unheard of in previous generations are striking modern societies around the world. At least thirty new diseases have emerged since Dr. Strachan began his work, and together they threaten the health of hundreds of millions around the world. If outbreaks of SARS, the West Nile Virus, Ebola, and COVID-19 weren't enough, how many people do you know who suffer from asthma, allergies of all kinds, irritable bowel syndrome, rheumatoid arthritis, lupus, Crohn's disease, chronic fatigue syndrome, or immune disorders of some kind? The list of what can go wrong in our bodies seems endless.

The answer doesn't lie in the stars but here on Earth with dirt—or to be more specific, the microbes in earth's soil. If we're to stay ahead of these deadly diseases, then dirt could be our new BFF. A report in New Scientist said researchers have discovered that microorganisms found in dirt influence the maturation of the immune system so that it is either functional or dysfunctional.

Long before the factories of the Industrial Age and the existence of modern grocery stores, people tended to get dirty by buying food at a farmer's market or working a garden plot in their backyard. We need to do more of that. The longest-lived people were exposed to all sorts of microscopic bugs living in the soil. Because life in the pre–Industrial Age depended on what grew and lived in and on the earth, "dirt" and "soil" were not negative concepts in the minds of our primitive ancestors.

Reward Offered: My Missing Microorganisms

Technology is certainly expanding exponentially, but our time in nature is not. Many "enlightened" parents do everything they can today to keep Junior from getting "dirty." The sad truth is, our environment is too clean! Immune cells that don't have adequate exposure to soil microbes tend to overreact when they do come into contact with them. Too many adults and children have been denied this much-needed exposure to soil microorganisms. Thus, their immune systems overreact because they are no longer being properly "educated" in the biological playground of life.

To make matters worse, we oversterilize everything with disinfectant dishwashing, hand soaps, shower gels, disinfectant body lotions, skin bars, and deodorant soaps loaded with antibiotic disinfectants such as triclosan. Furthermore, we sterilize our soil by using pesticides and herbicides that destroy beneficial and harmful microbes alike. These agents harm even the natural immune systems of the very plants that we're trying to "help" with our technological advances.

After years of medical and nutritional research, I'm convinced that our immune systems need regular exposure to naturally occurring soil organisms for long-term health. When the immune systems of children are deprived of early exposure to soil organisms, they may seriously overreact when exposed to various benign intruders later in life. It seems to be a consequence of our lost connection with earth that children and adults develop allergies, autoimmune diseases, and certain types of asthma.

That's why the best thing our family is doing is living part of the year on our Missouri farmland in the southern part of the state. Each day, our children are playing in the dirt, running through mounds of compost next to the chicken coops, picking up their share of dirty goats and chickens, and getting dusty from traveling around the ranch on our all-terrain vehicles.

Let me tell you—our kids are dirty at the end of the day and badly in need of a bath or shower. But that's a good thing because they were bathed by a shower of soil-based organisms through their close contact with dirt.

Th Cells: Equipped to Defend and Serve

A growing body of evidence implies the immune system will never reach its peak defensive capability against foreign organisms and chemical toxins until we reestablish this lost connection to the earth's soil.

Exposure to these microorganisms conditions the human immune system so that it intuitively knows when to produce and activate non-differentiated T-helper cells (Th cells) that are primarily produced by the thymus gland. These Th cells control the initiation or suppression of the body's immune reactions, and they also regulate many other immune cells. The quality and strength of the immune system are often measured with a classification method called the "Th1/Th2 balance."

Th1 cells promote specialized cell-mediated (meaning inside the cell) immunity. These are the quintessential "special forces" that defend the body efficiently. Th1 cells produce only as many germ-zapping antibodies as necessary to stop an invader. Theirs is a targeted response with economy of action.

Th2 cells, on the other hand, produce a mass response to infection in the form of specialized proteins called antibodies, secreted into body fluids by "B" cells (or B-lymphocytes). Th2 cells are the army and navy—the "total response" defenders in your body.

These two infection-fighting forces exist side by side. The body's Th1 cellular immunity force attacks abnormal cells and microorganisms at the site of infection—inside the individual cells. Th2 cells trigger the mass production of antibodies to neutralize foreign invaders and substances—outside the cells.

A healthy immune system has balanced Th1 and Th2 activity, and it can switch back and forth between the two as needed to eradicate a threat quickly. Illnesses result from immune system under response and overresponse. For example, the overabundance of Th2 antibodies is implicated in a wide variety of chronic illnesses, including AIDS, chronic fatigue syndrome, candidiasis, chronic allergies, multiple chemical sensitivities (MCS), viral hepatitis, cancer, lupus, and many other illnesses.

"Organisms 'R' Us"

The soil across the North American continent has been exceedingly rich in bacteria and other organisms for thousands of years, and every civilization—from nomadic Native American tribes to the early settlers—enjoyed the "amber waves of grain" that this land produced. The foods harvested from the field were covered with beneficial microorganisms that proved to be very beneficial to everyone who consumed these fresh-from-the-farm foodstuffs.

After World War II, however, a massive increase in pesticide usage by commercial agribusiness depleted many of the natural soil organisms on farms from Portland, Maine to Portland, Oregon. Year after year, decade after decade has only worsened the situation.

Today, America's soil is essentially sterile. At one time, pesticides and herbicides were believed to be the "total solution" in the natural world, but they also kill virtually every microorganism they touch—meaning healthy microorganisms are destroyed as well. Away from farmlands, our overuse of medical antibiotics has reduced the human gut to a burned-out minefield, destroying the good guys along with the bad guys.

As I've stated, most people aren't exposed to large enough quantities of microorganisms from our soil, dust, air, water, and foods to achieve optimal health on a daily basis. These days, you have to work or live on a farm or work with animals like a veterinarian to take in large amounts of beneficial microorganisms, either through dirt on the hands or involuntarily breathing in animal dung when exposed to large herds of livestock.

I know of one veterinarian in the Midwest who spends most of his time tending large herds of livestock in barns, feeding areas, and fields. His immune system is like iron, and he very rarely suffers from colds or the usual respiratory complaints because of his exposure to a wide variety of microorganisms.

For most of us, however, our overly sterile environment has seriously weakened our immune systems. And the sterility of our foods isn't helping our immune systems either. We have learned to increase shelf life by irradiating or chemically treating our produce and prepared foods to kill microorganisms. These modern, high-tech processing methods used by food manufacturers remove and destroy many of the important life-giving nutrients in our food.

Drinking an Indiscriminate Killer

Water supplies from wells and rivers once teemed with mycobacteria, including some pathogens that were downright deadly. Chlorine and other disinfectant substances have helped make our public water supplies much safer than a century ago, which is undoubtedly important to public health. Unfortunately, most municipal water purification systems neglect to remove the chlorine after the bleaching agent has done its job in the water.

The chlorine we ingest wipes out all bacteria—even the "good guys" inside our bodies. We're drinking an indiscriminate killer with the government's blessing, which is why I recommend filtering your tap water with a high-quality purification system to remove the chlorine.

Did You Get Your RDA of Antibiotics?

We have discussed the problem of treating symptoms of disease with antibiotics, because they kill both good and bad bacteria. Even if you don't take antibiotics, you almost certainly consume them in animal products. United States pharmaceutical firms produce more than 35 million pounds of antibiotics each year, and animals receive the vast bulk of them. Growers routinely give big helpings of antibiotics to cattle, pigs, and poultry to prevent infections from spreading in their stressful, crowded quarters. The situation is so bad that the European Union refuses to import livestock from American farms.

Researchers estimate that by consuming just one glass of commercially processed and packaged milk from your local supermarket shelf, you unknowingly ingest the residues of as many as one hundred different antibiotics. (Perhaps these little critters should be included in the government's official RDA list of "Recommended Daily Allowances.") This constant exposure to low-dose antibiotics is one reason behind the increase in antibiotic-resistant bacteria.

The intestines of healthy children and adults normally contain billions of bacteria and up to 10,000 different species of microorganisms. Ideally, the beneficial or benign bacteria in your body should outnumber the cells of your body by approximately one hundred to one. One side benefit of these friendly bacteria is that they also increase the body's levels of interferon, a powerful immunity-boosting chemical. These beneficial bacteria are your best friends!

Handling the Double-edged Sword

The beneficial bacteria in the environment and in your gut serve as your first line of immune defense against the unfriendly bacteria and fungi without and within. This is the "doubled-edged sword" of hygiene: while you want to keep your immune system from being overloaded with harmful substances, you also want to be exposed to the environment enough to "set" and properly program your immune responses for maximum effectiveness.

Adults and children face even more problems in our toxic world when stress, medications, and poor diet combine to reduce friendly bacteria to such a great extent that unfriendly bacteria begin to thrive. That is exactly what happens when high doses of antibiotics wipe out all the bacteria in your gut.

Once that happens, the race is on to see whether the "good guys" or the "bad guys" recolonize and set up shop in the empty real estate of a sterile digestive system. Unfortunately, if the harmful bacteria gain the upper hand (as they usually do because they thrive on a sugary, high-carbohydrate diet), poor health often results.

Get Your Gut Balanced and Get Well

The best way to quickly replenish and stabilize friendly bacteria in the gastrointestinal tract and develop a balanced immune system that reacts only as needed is the regular ingestion of live, fermented, probiotic-rich food and supplementation with homeostatic soil organisms. Soil-based organisms (SBOs), in addition to a diet that includes liberal amounts of cultured or fermented foods such as yogurt, kefir, and sauerkraut, will create the proper balance that your gut needs to be healthy.

Soil-based organisms produce proteins that the body interprets as antigens, which are proteins from a foreign substance or microorganism that stimulate an immune response. The way the soil organisms stimulate the Th cells of the immune system directly influences other immune cells, especially the B-lymphocytes manufactured in the bone marrow. Together, they trigger production of nonspecific or unprogrammed antibodies.

Unprogrammed antibodies have not been preprogrammed to overreact to foreign substances. They remain free and available for specific assignment to points of the body where they are needed. Constant exposure to soil organisms helps to reeducate the body's Th cells so they become more tolerant of foreign cells, helping them to mount only necessary immune responses without excess. It is as if the SBOs send the immune cells "back to school" to learn their jobs all over again and perform them even better.

Regular ingestion of SBOs produces a significant reservoir of extra antibodies ready for targeted response, greatly increasing the effectiveness of an individual's immune system. (Unfortunately, this reservoir appears to diminish when SBO ingestion ends.) It seems that soil-based organisms can help restore the lost link between the human body and the earth.

Several years after I made my health comeback in San Diego, I met a board-certified gastroenterologist named Joseph Brasco, M.D., who was seeking new options for his patients with gastrointestinal disorders. Dr. Brasco had read about my recovery from Crohn's disease in the magazine story published in the Townsend Letter for Doctors and Patients about how soil-based organisms played a huge role in my health comeback. He began recommending SBO supplementation to his patients and witnessed startling health turnarounds. We hit it off when we met and became close friends. Prior to writing the original Maker's Diet, Dr. Joe and I joined forces to co-author Restoring Your Digestive Health because of we both wanted to help those suffering from digestive problems.

Reverse the Vicious Cycle

Unfortunately, as Dr. Brasco can attest from dealing with thousands of patients over the years, people who are sick or who are recovering from a sickness tend to seek out comfort foods such as pizza, parmesan bread, hoagie sandwiches, milk shakes, cookies, and ice cream. These are the very foods that promote the rapid growth of disease-causing bacteria! This dysbiosis, or bacterial imbalance in the gut, results in abnormal fermentation in the small intestine.

Fermentation is somewhat desirable in the large intestine because it produces butyrate and other short-chain fatty acids that nourish the cells of the intestinal wall. In the small intestine, however, the growth of yeast, fungi, and/or fermenting pathogenic bacteria may damage the gut lining and cause toxic byproducts to be absorbed, which can impair the absorption of vital nutrients.

Instead of eating junk food and feeding the vicious cycle, you can improve the microbial balance in your gut by consuming the nutrient-rich live foods in the Maker's Diet as well as nutritional supplements with SBOs.

Antibiotic Bandages Cover More Serious Issues

Individuals who make repeated use of broad-spectrum antibiotics, oral con-traceptives, and steroid medications may set up conditions for the overgrowth of opportunistic organisms in their bodies that can recolonize rapidly once antibiotic treatment has ended, causing more disease symptoms. In a way, excessive antibiotic treatments become temporary bandages placed over more serious health issues with far-reaching consequences.

In short, it could be easier to treat symptoms than to do the extensive med-ical sleuthing it often takes to get to the root cause of patients' complaints. Medical science routinely resorts to antibiotics to deal with recognized symp-toms, but that form of medical treatment doesn't assure the elimination or the cause of those symptoms.

Yeast and fungal organisms are especially aggressive in weakened intestinal systems. When antibiotics kill the harmful bacteria they are targeting, as well as the friendly bacteria in the body, this allows other harmful bacteria that are normally held in check by the friendly bacteria to begin to multiply profusely, causing other disease conditions.

For example, the overgrowth of Candida albicans, an especially potent yeast-like fungus, can lead to a potentially serious condition called candidi-asis that results in the inflammation of the tongue, mouth, rectum, or vagina (in female patients), or trigger a range of mental and emotional symptoms, including irritability, anxiety, and even depression. Many allergies have been causally linked to Candida yeast overgrowth, which sometimes goes unde-tected because symptoms initially may appear to be innocuous digestive disorders such as bloating, heartburn, constipation, and diarrhea.

Secret Abuse at the Pharmacy

The abuse of antibiotic medication often starts with our children. According to the American Academy of Pediatrics, 95 percent of the children in the United States will receive treatment with antibiotics for a middle ear infec-tion by age five. Most children will tolerate it, but others will not fare as well once the antibiotics destroy their population of beneficial bacteria.

Research has shown that the prevention and treatment of dysbiosis and dysbacteriosis are among the most challenging problems doctors face today!

When dysbiosis sets in, creating imbalance between the protective bacteria and the unfriendly bacteria, even normally harmless organisms may produce illness.

Studies implicate intestinal bacterial imbalances as a basis for conditions ranging from recurrent infections and immune breakdown to chronic fatigue. Dysbiosis may leave you predisposed to ailments such as diarrhea, constipation, irritable bowel syndrome, colon cancer, allergies, vaginitis, increased susceptibility to infection, food cravings, lack of mental clarity, hypoglycemia, and many more conditions. Most doctors would rarely connect the cause of these illnesses to the microbial populations of the gastrointestinal tract.

Gut Problems Are Only the Beginning

Dysbiosis, which is the imbalance of microorganisms in the gut, may also affect body tissues far from the intestinal site, including the brain, joints, muscles, and immune system. Dysbiosis has a way of "exporting their misery" very effectively. Symptoms are diverse and may include headaches, learning disorders, insomnia, immune dysfunction, behavioral disorders, chronic fatigue, joint pain, and nutritional deficiencies.

Other more familiar conditions can also be traced to an imbalanced gastrointestinal tract microbial population. These include irritable bowel syndrome, Crohn's disease, fibromyalgia, leaky gut syndrome, wasting disease, diverticulitis, hemorrhoids, and breast and colon cancer.

Where the Gut Hits the Wallet

Contrary to the popular notion that ignorance is bliss, at least where your health is concerned, ignorance can be costly at best and deadly at worst. Digestive diseases and other conditions related to unhealthy intestinal flora imbalances in the gut have an enormous impact on our health and the nation's financial bottom line as well. Intestinal flora refers to a complex of microorganism species that live in the digestive tract.

New technologies and new drugs have revolutionized the understanding and treatment of peptic ulcer disease and gastrointestinal esophageal reflux disease (GERD). Everyone hopes that future research will reduce the economic and health-care costs related to diagnosing and treating digestive diseases. But I believe we could benefit right now by tapping proven wisdom from the past.

Your body desperately requires healthy intestinal flora because your health depends on it. A healthy gastrointestinal system has a balance of approximately 85 percent good bacteria to 15 percent bad microorganisms. Unfortunately, most of us show the reverse ratio. My own nearly fatal struggle with Crohn's disease was a severe example of what can happen when microbial imbalance abounds. If our ignorance about hygiene contributes to the problem, then we should determine to educate ourselves. The benefits we reap will be immense.

The following chart summarizes the simple steps you can take to restore and maintain a healthy gut.

STEPS TO A HEALTHY GUT
1.   Restore your connection to the soil.
• You may not be comfortable making mud pies, so I recommend that you do a little gardening, hike in the mountains, or supplement your diet with homeostatic soil organisms. A growing number of scientists, nutritionists, and medical doctors are convinced this is the most effective way to enhance the healing response of the body.
2.   Reap the benefits of HSO supplementation.
• Most people who begin HSO supplementation in concert with healthy dietary choices see a rapid and overall improvement in bodily functions and natural immunity to disease and infection.
3.   Know that SBOs can act as a protective shield.
• Soil organisms also produce substances called *bacteriocins*, which act as natural antibiotics to kill almost any kind of pathogenic microorganisms and to set up a protective shield in the gut. Hardy SBOs can survive the harsh environment of the gut. Unlike traditional probiotics, SBOs seem to be much hardier and are better able to survive the harsh environment of the intestine until they reach the location where they are most needed in the gut.
4.   Use SBOs to flush unfriendly microorganisms out of the body.
• Soil organisms seem to be especially well equipped to establish colonies in the entire digestive system, starting in the esophagus and ending in the colon. They attach themselves to the walls of the digestive tract and burrow behind any putrefaction lining the intestinal walls, where they consume or destroy unfriendly microorganisms. The waste products are then dislodged and flushed out of the body in the normal evacuation process.

STEPS TO A HEALTHY GUT
5.   Realize that SBOs obliterate yeast and molds.

- SBOs also seem to act aggressively against protozoa, worms, and other parasites within the intestines and related organs and tissues. Even *Candida albicans,* along with other yeast and molds, is obliterated.

Do You Need an Immune Boost?

The natural detoxification of the intestinal tract promoted by SBOs increases the body's ability to absorb nutrients. It also strengthens the immune system by removing mucoid plaque that covers the gut-associated lymphoid tissues (GALT), and it boosts the body's ability to fight off infectious viruses and bacteria.

If these statements sound a little far-fetched, remember that scientists from the world's leading research institutions, governmental health agencies, and pharmaceutical firms are scouring the soils of the earth for more soil organisms from which to create their medicines. The following list briefly describes the health benefits that scientists attribute to the consumption of soil-based organisms:

- **Pool new RNA/DNA in the cells.** SBOs provide a rich source of coded instructions for the cells to reactivate their own repair called DNA and RNA. SBOs appear to work in a symbiotic (mutually beneficial) relationship with body tissues by creating a pool of extra DNA/RNA raw materials. This reserve is immediately available upon demand, accelerating the healing process when cells are damaged by wounds, burns, surgical incisions, and infections.

- **Quench free radicals by creating superoxide dismutase (SOD).** SBOs produce superoxide dismutase (SOD), a powerful antioxidant. Unless extinguished at once, free radicals attack any physiological molecule, causing cancers and other tissue damage. SOD works enzymatically as a first-line defense against free radicals, stopping them cold before they can cause organ damage.

- **Stimulate alpha interferon production.** SBOs seem to stimulate the production of the polypeptide alpha interferon (a molecular protein and a key immune system regulator). The scientific community long ago recognized the virus-fighting ability of alpha interferon. They synthesized the alpha interferon to treat a variety of illnesses, including hepatitis C.

- **Stimulate the production of human lactoferrin.** A substance present in homeostatic soil organisms stimulates the formation of human lactoferrin, one of the body's iron-carrying proteins. The iron carried by the lactoferrin protein is released to healthy cells and not available to feed pathogenic microorganisms or contribute to iron overload.

The newly recognized ability of soil organisms to aid our quest for healing and maintaining good health is one of the most exciting breakthroughs in modern health. And isn't it ironic that we are talking about soil organisms as old as the earth?

I would urge anyone with intractable autoimmune conditions, allergies, low energy, inability to gain weight, fibromyalgia, and chronic fatigue syndrome to take advantage of SBOs. Parents of children with chronic middle ear infections would do well by their children to give them SBO supplementation as well.

HOW TO KNOW IF YOU HAVE DYSBIOSIS	*Dysbiosis* is a health condition of living with intestinal flora that has harmful effects, due to putrefaction, fermentation (carbohydrate intolerance), deficiency, or sensitization. The following lists include many of the symptoms and major causes of dysbiosis.

Common symptoms are:

- abdominal pain or cramps
- colon cancer
- constipation or diarrhea
- distention/bloating
- fatigue/fatigue after eating
- flatulence (excessive gas)
- bad breath
- body odor
- food allergy
- hypoglycemia

- inability to lose weight
- irregular bowel movements
- irritable bowel syndrome
- itchy anus
- leaky gut syndrome
- poor complexion
- poor digestion
- rheumatoid arthritis
- spastic colon

Major causes are:

- decreased immune function
- decreased intestinal motility (constipation)
- drugs—especially antibiotics, oral contra-ceptives, and cortisone-like medications
- intestinal infection
- maldigestion and malabsorption
- poor diet from excessive carbohydrates, sugar, and trans fats
- stress, including long-term emotional stress

Will You Choose a Road Less Traveled?

Even though they were virtually unknown just two hundred years ago, we now know that these invisible organisms, good and bad, play vital roles in our health—and, potentially, in our destruction.

In this chapter, I have discussed three simple steps to guard our health from the bad guys and strengthen it with the good guys:

1. First, we balance the double-edged sword of hygiene by cleansing rather than sterilizing our bodies (particularly under the fingernails and around the eyes and nasal passages) using advanced hygiene. This permits exposure to the environment without overload.

2. Second, we feed our bodies healthy living foods from the Maker's Diet.

3. Third, we repopulate and strengthen the living environment in the gut with SBOs.

These are three relatively simple steps to improved health. Most of us, however, are careening down a different path, following what I call the "modern prescription for illness." This is an easily accessible path of least resistance that comes through following the standard American diet (SAD), consuming whatever you find at America's fast-food restaurants, and filling your homes and bodies with toxic chemicals hidden in common items that advertisements make you believe you can't live without.

The destination is the same for all travelers—illness that could be avoided by taking a road less traveled, as I'll discuss in my next chapter.

≈

5

How to Get Sick:
A Modern Prescription for Illness

U NDER IDEAL CONDITIONS, EVERYONE WOULD BE BORN PERFECT AND
without flaws. In reality, we all carry genetic and metabolic weaknesses
and are bombarded by potentially harmful bacteria, viruses, fungi, and
industrial toxins around the clock. I'm convinced that we all have predetermined weaknesses in our bodies. Mine was the gut, but yours may be the
lungs, the cardiovascular system, the blood, or the kidneys.

If you eat unhealthy foods and adopt an unwise lifestyle, you may well see
these predetermined weaknesses present themselves with devastating effects.
Unfortunately, many of us exist in a state of sub-clinical illness, often unaware
of how unhealthy we really are. Whatever our state of health is, we can't afford
to go through life without taking certain precautions.

In my case, I have been taking extra care with my diet and lifestyle for the
last twenty years because I don't want a replay of my illness ever again. Ever
since I was cured, I have resisted taking medications of any kind—especially
antibiotics. And unless I'm forced at gunpoint, I will never knowingly take
another vaccination.

How to Get Sick

While I focus extensively on making wise food and dietary decisions elsewhere in this book, in this chapter I want to examine a short list of non-dietary
danger areas that may threaten your long-term health. In fact, if you want to
get sick, then all you have to do is follow a handful of these twenty-seven

recommendations—or maybe just one. But if you want to remain healthy as long as possible, go against all twenty-seven suggestions, if at all possible.

The list may surprise you. Be sure to examine the evidence and reasoning for each item to see why it made the dubious list I've called "How to Get Sick":

1. Stay out of the sun.

Civilizations throughout history have understood that the sun is vital to human health. The human skin uses the energy from the sun to manufacture vitamin D for the body. This hormone/vitamin is important for many reasons, including its role in strengthening immune system function and proper mineral absorption.

Critics claim that exposure to the UV rays of the sun cause higher rates of melanoma and other forms of skin cancer. This might be true for a small population segment—including those with compromised immune systems who don't consume adequate nutrients (especially healthy fats). People who actually get the most exposure to sunlight in different parts of the world, however, exhibit the lowest incidence of skin cancer. The only logical explanation is that exposure to sunlight is not unhealthy.

What's unhealthy is exposure to sunlight with the diets we consume. Rex Russell, M.D., noted that when sunlight activates the phytochemicals in healthy foods, consumption of these foods not only blocks the harmful effects of UV rays, but they also produce "antiviral, antibacterial, and anticancer components, as well as pest repellents."

2. Go to bed after midnight.

Looking for another great way to get sick? Try going to bed at 1 or 2 in the morning. From biblical times to just before the Industrial Revolution, people used to go to sleep and rise with the setting and rising of the sun. This was the natural way to link your peak activity to the body's natural hormonal rhythms.

The invention of the electric light changed all that, and these days it seems like people are going to bed later and later. A study published in The Lancet (a respected medical journal in Great Britain) indicated that chronic sleep loss produces serious symptoms mimicking the effects of aging and the early stages of diabetes—including age-related insulin resistance and memory loss.

3. Never let them see you sweat.

Any attempt to artificially prevent perspiration is unhealthy because perspiration is the Maker's method of safely cooling the body while excreting numerous toxins. Suppressing this natural sweat response in your underarms blocks the body's cleansing process and the natural flow of the lymphatic system. Interference in normal lymphatic function may increase the risk of breast cancer.

The products most often used to stop perspiration contain forms of:

* aluminum, which has been linked to Alzheimer's disease or other neurological problems
* triclosan, an antimicrobial absorbed through the skin that poses some risk to the liver
* zirconium-based compounds that can cause underarm granulomas

For more information about these products and possible alternative choices, see The Safe Shopper's Bible by David Steinman and Samuel S. Epstein, M.D.

4. Take megadoses of vitamins and minerals.

The use of massive amounts of over-the-counter vitamins and minerals can be harmful, especially if you take the popular and cheap synthetic and isolated "vitamins" created in chemical plants and widely sold in discount retail stores. The human body was not designed to consume such artificial products, especially in such excessive amounts. Nature prevents us from consuming 20,000 mg of vitamin C in one day because it is impossible to consume three hundred oranges (a natural source of vitamin C) in a twenty-four-hour timeframe.

But let's say you managed that feat. If so, that many oranges would produce one major colon cleanse! Vitamins and minerals that have not been incorpoo rated into an organic matrix—a natural food form containing all necessary co-factors—may actually be destructive to the body. It's better to supplement healthy food and beverage choices with living food supplements known as homeostatic nutrients rich in vitamins and minerals. This is a balanced form the body can absorb and utilize.

5. Use fluoride toothpaste and mouthwash twice a day, and be sure to drink a lot of fluoridated water.

Fluoride is extremely toxic—especially the salt-based form used in toothpaste and mouthwash. (Besides, its effectiveness is questionable at best.) A top EPA scientific advisor voiced the opinion that "since recent federal government tests have shown that fluoride appears to cause cancers at levels less than ten times the present maximum contamination level, this would ordinarily require that all additions of fluoride to water supplies be suspended and treatment be instituted to remove naturally occurring fluoride." That would be enough warning for me!

By the way, since the original Maker's Diet was released, I have no evidence that the EPA ever suspended fluoridation operations. Choose non-fluoridated alternatives for oral hygiene to be safe.

6. Use artificial sweeteners and avoid sugars.

As bad as sugar can be in its various forms, artificial sweeteners are worse. Some are downright deadly because of their carcinogenic properties and use in such high-volume products as diet soft drinks and sugar-free foods. Chief among sinners is aspartame, which is marketed as NutraSweet (the pink packets) or Equal (the blue packets).

Renowned diabetes expert Dr. H. J. Roberts believes there is a clear scientific link between aspartame and increased incidence of brain tumors, seizure disorders, chronic headaches, and hyperactivity in children. As for saccharin, the cancer-causing labels that accompany its use still apply. Ten years ago, the newcomer on the block was sucralose, which is available in those yellow packets of Splenda, but no matter what artificial sweetener is used, it's a horrible idea to drink beverages or consume foods filled with these long-alleged cancer risks.

7. Shower every day, but don't bathe (take a bath).

Excessive showering—even in the purest water—can rob your hair and body of natural oils and wash away beneficial microbes that are important to your gut health. "Good bacteria are educating your own skin cells to make your own antibiotics [and] they produce their own antibiotics that kills off bad bacteria," noted Dr. Richard Gallow, chief of the dermatology division at the University of California, San Diego.

By showering too often, you strip your skin of beneficial oils, which leads to dry, flaky skin and can worsen certain conditions like eczema. "It's not just removing the lipids and oils on your skin that's drying it out…it could be removing some of the good bacteria that help maintain a healthy balance of skin."

Standing a long time until a shower of warm water can also alter your body's pH, especially if you're using certain alkaline shampoos and soaps. That doesn't even account for the added problem of showering with heavily chlorinated public water (see below).

If the Maker has a preference, it might be the use of ritual bathing that combined bathing (washing in a shallow bath) with sprinkling (showering for brief periods). This combination is especially beneficial for the thorough but gentle cleansing recommended for the female genital area.

If you shower every day—which the average American does—you might want to skip washing your hair or lathering up every now and then to give your skin a break.

8. Swim in chlorinated pools, and be sure to drink and shower with chlorinated water.

Chlorine is an effective bacteria killer, although some strains of bacteria are developing a resistance to chlorine. Unfortunately, chlorine is an indiscriminate killer that kills both friendly and unfriendly bacteria. The chemical element also eats through lead pipes, corrodes most metals, and harms cells and DNA strands in virtually every living thing it touches. Chlorine also introduces highly carcinogenic chemicals called trihalomethanes (THMs) into our water supply.

Studies show a strong link between chlorinated water supplies with elevated THM levels and cancers of the bladder, kidney, liver, pancreas, gastrointestinal tract, urinary tract, colon, and brain. It's risky enough to drink chlorinated tap water, but the mass exposure created by swimming in chlorinated pools or taking extended hot showers in heavily chlorinated water is much more dangerous. (The heat opens skin pores and increases the already high absorption rate of chlorine through the skin.) Dogs exposed to chlorine—which, by the way, is also a bleaching agent in white bread—get the running fits, a disorder similar to many psychiatric disorders in humans.

9. Don't breastfeed your baby—feed him or her formula instead.

Mothers, don't consider breastfeeding your children if you want them to risk the trauma of numerous childhood diseases and if you want to pay their hospital bills. Don't breastfeed unless you want to reduce your risk of developing breast cancer by 25 percent and lower the risk of postpartum depression.

Actually, there's nothing better than mother's milk, which contains cells that attack harmful bacteria in the baby's system and is able to form antibodies that destroy invading viruses as well. Mother's milk is the Maker's perfect food for babies, delivered in the close bonds of maternal intimacy.

10. Get tattoos.

I understand that tattoos are quite popular today, even mainstream, but Scripture warns against piercing the skin. (See Leviticus 19:28.) Sure, we have freedom in Christ, but body piercing and tattoos easily introduce potentially deadly infections and toxic foreign substances into the body and bloodstream. Some health providers warn that even tiny puncture wounds might block important electrical nerve impulses just under the skin.

11. Get all of your immunization shots.

The topic of childhood immunizations, once dormant, is back in the news with measles outbreaks and remains as controversial as ever. That said, I believe certain childhood immunization injections may pose considerable risks to children.

If you were born before 1980, you probably received one to five immunizations in childhood, but schoolchildren today receive an average of twenty-two or more immunizations—most of them administered while the brain and nervous system are still developing! An epidemic of juvenile autism and other neurological and developmental disorders sweeping through America's school-age children has generally coincided with the introduction of certain mandatory immunizations.

Most states allow philosophical and religious exemptions from mandatory immunization programs should you decide this is the way to go. The decision to vaccinate or not to vaccinate your children is not one to take lightly and deserves your full attention.

12. Travel in airplanes often.

I've only gotten sick a handful of times since I wrote *The Maker's Diet*, but I bet I could trace each event to a plane flight I took. Being trapped in a flying tube at 39,000 feet with a couple hundred sneezing, coughing people is almost a surefire guarantee to catch a nasty bug that your body can't beat back.

The bathrooms on airplanes have always been problematic, at least for me, because they are flying germ farms. San Diego State biology professor Scott Kelley took a small but scientific sampling of airline cleanliness several years ago when participants swabbed surfaces at ten different places aboard various flights. They took biological evidence not only from armrests and tray tables, but toilet seats and handles, sinks, floors, unused paper towels, and doorknobs coming in and out of the planes' bathrooms.

The good professor said the results were what you'd expect from a fraternity house. He discovered opportunistic pathogens like Streptococcus, Staphylococcus, Cornybacterium, Proprionibacterium, and Kocuria. Kelley said the situation doesn't warrant wearing surgical gloves the next time you board a flight, but he mentioned that whenever he flies and uses the facilities, he washes his hands well and uses a paper towel to open the lavatory door as he leaves. I've opened more lavatory doors with a paper towel than I care to count, and you should, too. The bathroom knob was the nastiest part of the plane, Scott Kelley said.

Aircraft cabins are pressurized to an altitude of 8,000 feet; some people who spend a lot of time at high altitudes like that experience problems with infertility and oxygen production in the body. The body adapts well to high altitudes for short periods of time, but not for long periods.

Some researchers believe the atmospheric pressures and radiation to which airplane travelers are exposed are the equivalent of hundreds of CAT scans and pose the greatest oxidative stress on the human body.

13. Expose yourself often to electromagnetic energy.

Everywhere you go, you run into electromagnetic fields (EMFs) from television sets, microwave ovens, cell phones, and local media transmission towers. Studies conducted over the last two decades imply possible association of EMFs with miscarriages, birth defects, leukemia, brain cancers, breast cancers, and lymphomas. Hospital body scans (X-rays and their computerized

cousins, computerized axial tomography [CAT scans]) and magnetic reso-
nance imaging (MRI) expose us to especially high levels of EMFs.

One MRI delivers radiation equal to one hundred conventional X-rays.
Cellular phones may pose dangers to brain tissues due to the close proximity
of delicate brain tissue to powerful EMF transmitters. The good news is that
most EMF exposure can be avoided or limited because it occurs in the home
through the use of electric blankets, microwave ovens, hair dryers, television
sets, and computers.

Avoid getting too close to these devices while in use. Use regular blankets
instead of electric ones, and make sure all appliances and electrical instal-
lations in your home are in working order with all protective devices and
protocols in place. As for microwave ovens, they are problematic, and we don't
have one in the home.

14. Use a lot of skin care products, cosmetics, hair care products, nail care products, shampoos, soaps, perfumes, shaving cream, suntan lotion, and antibacterial soaps.

Beware of skin care products that cause harm by destroying the skin's natural pH through the introduction of dangerous toxins to the body. Hair-coloring
products used by approximately 40 percent of U.S. women, particularly brown
and black hair products, are associated with increased incidence of Hodgkin's
lymphoma, multiple myeloma, Hodgkin's disease, and 20 percent of all
non-Hodgkin's lymphoma. (There are several brands of natural hair-coloring
products that are relatively safe.)

Also avoid products containing DEA or TEA—these ingredients often contain carcinogenic nitrosamine impurities. Toluene, a neuro-toxic substance
that triggers asthma attacks and causes asthma in previously unaffected
people, was found in every fragrance sample tested by the EPA in 1991. The
fragrance industry routinely uses hundreds and hundreds of toxic substances.
As for shampoos, many of the most common ingredients break down into
formaldehyde. For detailed information on things to avoid and where to find
good alternatives, see The Safe Shopper's Bible and Diet for a Poisoned Planet.

As for antibacterial soaps, most of them contain triclosan, which may be
absorbed through the skin and pose a risk to the liver. Plenty of regular soap,

sufficiently heated running water, and thorough scrubbing will do the job just as well. Advanced hygiene is the best cleansing plan I've found to date.

15. Take lots of medications.

Every medicine has a side effect. There's a time and place for the use of medications, but much of the prescription activity in the U.S. perpetuates health problems by treating symptoms rather than their root causes.

Medications such as antibiotics, oral contraceptives, and corticosteroids may cause major problems with the gastrointestinal terrain, damage the immune system, cause liver problems, and alter enzyme function. The practice of taking a baby aspirin each day to prevent heart attacks is one I don't recommend, for instance. Aspirin can cause bleeding in the intestinal track and be toxic to the liver.

You can get similar health benefits with no side effects by consuming foods in the Maker's Diet such as cold-1

16. Get your cavities filled with mercury.

For more than 150 years, the dental profession has carefully avoided using the term mercury when describing the material used to fill tooth cavities for millions of Americans. They called it "silver amalgam," "silver fillings," or "amalgam fillings." The true composition of dental amalgam is 45 to 55 percent mercury, with about 30 percent silver and other metals such as copper, tin, and zinc.

Mercury is a heavy metal toxin. According to BioProbe, an independent non-profit watchdog agency, vapor released continuously from mercury amalgam fillings in your mouth can produce "neurological and psychiatric symptoms... such as depression, irritability, exaggerated response to stimulation, excessive shyness, insomnia, emotional instability, forgetfulness, confusion, and vasomotor disturbances such as excessive perspiration and uncontrolled blushing. Tremors are also common in individuals exposed to mercury vapor."

The organization cites one estimate that approximately "26 million amalgam bearers whose allergies may be causally related to their mercury/amalgam dental fillings" would benefit by replacing mercury amalgam fillings with safer alternative materials. It may be difficult to find a dentist in your area who will fill your cavities with more natural materials, but it isn't impossible.

The movement continues to grow despite significant opposition from the American Dental Association and state dental boards.

17. Do aerobic exercise.

While I believe strongly in the need for regular exercise, my research indicates that high-intensity exercise producing a high, elevated heart rate for long periods of time through vigorous exercises such as jogging or running on hard surfaces is unnatural to the body. You should exercise as the body was designed to by incorporating the principles of functional fitness. Typically, human beings in virtually every culture have engaged in the anaerobic type of functional exercise common to regular labor or work functions on the farm, on the water, or while hunting wild game.

Long-distance walking or slower-paced labor functions may have been punctuated by intense but relatively brief bursts of physical labor or high-speed movement. Intense aerobic exercise supports immune response and creates more oxidation through stress than anaerobic exercise (strength training).

18. Wear contact lenses and receive silicone breast implants.

Breast implants are popular, widely advertised, and admired in today's culture, but no one talks about the long-term or short-term risks of planting a foreign object into the body. Women can choose from two kinds of breast implants:

- saline implants are filled with a saline or saltwater solution
- silicone implants are filled with silicone gel

During the 1980s, when silicone breast implants were the rage, more and more women reported that their implants ruptured. Lawsuits were filed, and women complained of immunological disorders such as fibromyalgia and rheumatoid arthritis. The Food and Drug Administration banned silicone breast implants in 1992, but in 2006, the agency reversed course and approved the sale of certain types of silicone implants.

Suddenly, plastic surgeons got very busy because women prefer the look and feel of silicone implants over the saline version. Even though breast implants have never been more popular than they are today, the risk of rupture and leakage means women are putting their health at risk—needlessly so, in my opinion. (I'm referring to women who seek out breast augmentation to increase the size of their bust, not those who lost their breasts from mastectomy surgery and are seeking reconstructive surgery.)

My issue with contact lenses, especially the soft lens variety offered for long-term wear, is that they pose significant infection risks to the wearers under certain conditions. While contacts offer certain conveniences and cosmetic benefits, remember that they are still foreign substances that the Maker never intended for us to insert into the human body. I'm convinced that contacts pose risks to our immune systems.

19. Live in a home with toxic paint, toxic carpet, toxic mold, and toxic paraffin candles, etc.

You could fill a small library with the books and official research reports written on this subject. Do some research if you or your family suffer from allergies or unexplained physical symptoms. Many popular building materials, including plywood, particle board, treated lumber, adhesives, paint, paint thinners, insulation, paint strippers, carpets, and carpet pads—even decorative paraffin candles—contain highly toxic materials such as formaldehyde, chloroform, lead vapor, arsenic, and countless other toxins. They can enter your living area as gaseous vapors and increase the toxic load of the body. Add to that the problem of toxic black molds, and you have a very toxic home.

20. Wear synthetic fabrics.

The Maker's natural fibers produce the ideal clothing for the human body. Such natural fibers as wool and cotton are far better to wear because they "breathe" and are better suited to handling human perspiration while preserving balanced body temperatures in hot or cold climates. Synthetic fibers often come from petroleum-based resins and other unnatural sources. Unfortunately, even conventionally grown cotton is often contaminated with numerous pesticides and chemical dyes.

21. Breathe with shallow breaths.

The Maker gave you two lungs with an amazing air capacity.

Unfortunately, most of us use only a fraction of our lung capacity and suffer for it. While infants are instinctive "belly breathers," most of us have learned to breathe by taking in short, shallow breaths that resemble a pant more than a deep breath.

The body—and the brain and nervous system in particular—thrives on abundant oxygen. Proper breathing relieves stress and lowers blood pressure, so breathe from the abdomen or "belly" instead of from the chest. If your stomach moves outward when you take a deep breath (and any breath for that matter), then you have learned the secret of breathing fully from the diaphragm.

22. Swallow your food without chewing well—or inhale your food as fast as you can.

Chewing is extremely important to proper digestion. The chewing reflex signals the body to release saliva containing the salivary enzyme ptyalin, a form of amylase, which begins to break down carbohydrates. Parotid glands behind the ears signal the thymus gland to produce T cells, just in case the food contains toxins or pathogens. The ultimate goal of the process is to deliver food to the stomach in a liquid state.

I'm convinced that my habit of "wolfing down" food in huge bites contributed to the development of Crohn's disease in my body. Horace Fletcher, who lived in the early 1900s, had an affliction known as Addison's disease, which produced major digestive problems and weight loss. Mr. Fletcher allegedly cured himself by chewing each mouthful of food thirty-five to fifty times. His story inspired others to be chewing their food thoroughly; they called themselves "Fletcherizers."

Since I've become a slow-chew kind of guy, don't go calling yourself a "Rubinizer." I recommend, however, chewing each bite twenty-five to fifty times as needed—especially when eating foods high in carbohydrates such as grains, sugars, and starches.

A last bit of advice: always eat sitting down and avoid watching TV, arguing, or doing something that requires concentration.

23. Use plastic food storage products, popular food wraps, and re-use plastic drinking bottles.

Plastic products release or leach carcinogenic toxins into foods. The toxicity is increased when foods contain high amounts of water or when they are highly acidic.

Water is one of nature's most effective solvents, and it is effective at drawing out toxins from plastic. The plastic in water bottles and baby bottles can leach BPA (bisphenol A) and other phthalates into liquids and foods. Seek out BPA- and phthalate-free bottles as well as glass containers, which are the safest containers of all.

If you happen to reuse plastic water bottles, be aware that researchers say repeated washing and reuse of disposable water bottles may accelerate the breakdown of the plastic, increasing your exposure to potentially harmful chemicals. Do not use plastic water bottles more than twice at the most.

As for aluminum foil, if you didn't already know that it's bad, then you know now. Some aluminum inevitably leaches into foods it touches, so when it comes to food storage, ditch aluminum wrap in favor of using glass Pyrex dishes and an environmentally safe plastic wrap that's PVC and plasticizer-free.

24. Eat grocery store produce and processed foods treated with pesticides, herbicides, animal growth hormones, and antibiotics; don't forget hybridized, irradiated, and GMO or genetically altered foods.

What a mouthful—literally! Pesticides and herbicides comprise one of the world's most deadly classes of chemical compounds. If a pesticide or herbicide kills one thing, it will probably kill, mutate, or seriously damage a whole host of other things.

The problem with these compounds is that they tend to stay on the fruit, vegetable, or plant they were applied to. Then there is the cumulative effect of adding the toxins from our water, air, food, and building materials year after year. Animal growth hormones don't go away after an animal is butchered, prepared for market, or cooked. They go right into our stomachs and continue their work. Nor do they disappear from the milk of a cow treated with antibiotics.

It is estimated that one glass of commercial, nonorganic milk purchased from a grocery story may contain the residue of up to one hundred antibiotics! Many of the meats we eat come from animals fed antibiotic-laden feeds. Growth hormones in our food supply are blamed for causing the abnormally early menses of young girls and for the overabundance of female hormones in young men. (Female hormones are given to milk cows to increase milk production.)

Most pesticides are known carcinogens, and some of them pose as counterfeit versions of the female hormone estrogen. These xenoestrogens may promote cancer by stimulating estrogen receptors in the body.

Hybridized foods are also very unhealthy with potentially deadly side effects. God says to eat every seed-bearing plant after its own kind, but hybridized, seedless watermelons or grapes cannot reproduce, so they may not be the healthy food sources you think they are. GMO or genetically modified foods are problematic, and irradiated foods—meaning microwaved—offer many of the same problems and dangers as other forms of radiation.

The government may reassure us they are safe, but the same government put U.S. soldiers at risk back in 1945 by encouraging them to stand out in the open and watch the early tests of the atomic bomb—with disastrous results. Of course, those soldiers were assured that they were totally safe.

25. Wear tight underclothing.

The body's lymph system is absolutely crucial to the immune system and is the first line of defense against cancer cells, toxins, and viral and bacterial attacks. Lymph nodes that are compressed or blocked by tight underclothing such as push-up bras, bustiers, or corsets may not allow the lymph system to be properly cleansed. For this reason, women shouldn't wear bras to bed.

26. Undergo surgery to remove "unnecessary body parts."

No one knows how many children fell victim to the medical myth common years ago that it was best to remove the tonsils to ensure the child wouldn't get tonsillitis. Parents were told by their doctors that the tonsils served no useful purpose anyway.

This myth has since been disproved and discarded, but other equally arrogant myths persist about the supposedly useless appendix, an appendage that "lost its purpose in the process of evolution somewhere." The truth is that the appendix and the tonsils are lymphoid tissues that aren't as unnecessary as some doctors may say.

Here's where I come down: It some part of your body was there when you were born, chances are your Maker intended for it to stay there until you die. Besides, there are risks every time you agree to enter a hospital for surgery. I'm talking about the risk of infection, surgical error, surgical complications, or dangerous drug interactions that may be far greater than the health problems you face outside of the hospital.

27. Visit your medical doctor often.

While I am thankful for all of the wonderful medical breakthroughs and excellent emergency medical care available in this country, you might want to know that according to a study by researchers at Johns Hopkins Medicine, medical errors are the third leading cause of death in the U.S., causing 250,000 deaths every year.

Dr. Barbara Starfield of the Johns Hopkins School of Hygiene and Public Health noted that a quarter of a million deaths occur each year due to a physician's activity, manner, or therapy. She was referring to 12,000 unnecessary surgeries, 7,000 medication errors in hospitals, 20,000 "other errors" in hospitals, 80,000 infections acquired in hospitals, and 106,000 "non-error, negative effects of drugs." (And these are the low estimates.)

Furthermore, the United States healthcare system is the most expensive in the world but ranks among eleven "First World" countries: Australia, Canada, France, Germany, the Netherlands, New Zealand, Norway, Sweden, Switzerland, and the United Kingdom.

I have no axe to grind, I really don't. Most doctors are sincere, hard-working professionals who try to do their jobs well. My biggest beef is that the medical profession's answer to the vast majority of illness is to write a prescription. And the downward spiral continues and never seems to stop.

Don't wait until the day you are stricken with a severe sickness and debilitating pain. Act now to rid yourself of all twenty-seven prescriptions for illness by adopting the Maker's Diet as your lifestyle to a better life.

≈

6

The Desperate Search for Health

IF THERE'S ONE THING I'VE LEARNED OVER THE YEARS, IT'S THAT MILLIONS of middle-aged American moms and dads, college students, and even younger teens sense that something is terribly wrong with their health. They just don't know what to do about it.

Best-selling health books offer ever-changing "flavor of the month" fad diets, while the media blow like a leaf in the wind, breathlessly telling us to eat a certain food one day and to avoid it the next. A recent example is the U.S. government stating that it's okay to drink up to five cups of coffee per day. I thought caffeine wasn't good for you!

So how does an exhausted forty-two-year-old mother lose weight safely while finding the energy to keep up with a vanload of active teenagers and younger children? How does she get her woefully out-of-shape husband back in to the gym and help her mother overcome the painful bouts with arthritis and an embarrassing overactive bladder?

Most mothers know better than to take these questions to their local HMO or their busy family physician. Though moms may not have a wall filled with medical degrees, they do run long on common sense—because they have to. Something inside tells them that none of the small health "miracles" they hope for will come from a pill or a bottle—or from a man or woman in a white lab coat.

Philosophy of Conventional Medicine

Conventional medicine sends its troops into battle against disease armed with surgery, pharmaceuticals, and invasive therapies such as chemotherapy and radiation. Anything outside the ironclad realm of a knife, a pill, or an X-ray machine is considered voodoo or worse. The genuine desire to maintain health is simply beyond the scope of this "take two-tablets-and-call-me-in-the-morning" philosophy.

Though maintenance of health is mentioned often in the world of alternative medicine, the practical function of defining and preserving genuine good health is beyond the reach of most conventional medical doctors because of their consuming focus on medications and surgical approaches to treating disease. Most medical doctors totally exclude basic nutrition from their treatment plans. Indeed, this makes total sense because they have little educational background to do otherwise.

Thus, you're on your own. I say that rhetorically, of course, but if you have a mindset of being in charge of your health, then prevention is key. Warding off disease and maintenance of health do not begin in the emergency room or intensive care ward of a hospital; they start with the lifestyle choices you make every day.

Don't get me wrong. I'm thankful for the surgical expertise in the United States, but I'm convinced that if you follow the genuine biblical nutritional and lifestyle principles that make up the Maker's Diet, then you will largely remove the need for most of the work done in surgical suites—or visit your local pharmacy as often. Instead, America's surgeons can devote a lot more time and energy into their vital roles in trauma and emergency medicine for accidents and other special cases if millions like you take charge of your health.

Most physicians have little or no training in nutrition, so I wonder why many confidently tell their patients that their diet has nothing to do with their sickness—even patients like myself with severe bowel disorders! As a result, many people leave their physician's office with a prescription and a nagging feeling that their symptoms are "all in my head."

It's not all in your head. It's in how you act and how you live your life.

Priorities for Healthcare Are Changing

Ever since *The Maker's Diet* was released, I've witnessed a growing pushback among millions of people whose lifestyle-related conditions and growing chronic health problems were not addressed by modern medicine. Even when presented for treatment, their conditions did not respond to conventional medical protocols. Feeling as if they were kicked to the curb by a sometimes arrogant and rigid medical system, these people have turned in greater and greater numbers to complementary and alternative healthcare.

Though conventional medicine has declared war on cancer, heart disease, and other killer diseases, it's definitely losing these battles despite vast expenditures on research. Some might convincingly argue that conventional medicine—as it is currently practiced in the United States—is actually shooting itself (and us) in the foot.

One thing is for sure: Americans' use of complementary and alternative medicine is not going away. According to a National Institutes for Health survey released in 2015, U.S. adults are using alternative medicine methods 38 percent of the time—a number that's been growing slowly but steadily for decades. Typical therapies include acupuncture, chiropractic manipulation, homeopathic treatments, massages, Pilates, naturopathy, and yoga classes.

Essentially, the shortcomings of conventional medicine have sent many adults looking for options, but let me candidly tell you that many of these alternative treatments—such as biofeedback, hypnosis, and Qi gong—are as suspect as their conventional counterparts. Care must be taken to ascertain that an alternative approach to health care is scientifically based and fundamentally sound, as I will discuss shortly.

My feeling on this whole matter about conventional and alternative medicine is that if you adopt the Maker's Diet, you'll enjoy a lot less chance of ever needing emergency or trauma medical services. Remember the great saying: "An ounce of prevention is worth a pound of cure."

But as I discovered during my battle with a supposedly incurable disease, once you step outside of the relatively predictable world of conventional medh icine, you find yourself on a very unpredictable hamster wheel of alternative medicine. It's virtually impossible to wade through the hundreds of miracle diets, pills, potions, and health programs out there—and I do mean "out there."

Something inside us desperately longs to return to the health and active lifestyles we once enjoyed, which is why alternative therapies are so beguiling. Empty promises and flashy marketing campaigns aside, many of these alternative treatments are incredibly expensive, and some may actually endanger your health. I know from painful personal experience that people who are desperate to get well or to regain some measure of health grasp at every straw that offers hope. (Like being told by a well-meaning nutritionist to eat straw, which happened to me one time.)

Step-by-step programs offering inflated guarantees of success are the most perilous attractions. There is a tremendous temptation to plug in to any promising program that gives us an easy road map to follow. Everyone wants to believe testimonials from those who lost fifty pounds or a dozen inches off their waist or beat back diabetes and regained their health, but that's not how it goes.

With the Maker's Diet, I refuse to insult your intelligence with simplistic health maxims and ridiculous promises without explaining the functional basis for the health therapy and lifestyle changes you may choose to embrace after reading this book.

But before I have you examine the functional basis for the Maker's Diet, I'm going to briefly analyze some of the more popular health diets available today. Perhaps you've tried some of these already. For this synopsis, I will have something to say about each of the following:

- Standard American diet (or "SAD")
- vegetarian diet (the Genesis and Hallelujah diets)
- raw food diet
- anti-*Candida* diet
- balanced macronutrient ratios diet (the "Zone")
- ketogenic or "low-carb" diet (Atkins' and South Beach diets)
- food-combining diets
- blood-type diet

The Standard American Diet (SAD)

The "standard" American diet typically includes a doughnut or muffin with coffee and orange juice for breakfast followed by a midmorning bagel with cream cheese. Lunch is likely be a turkey sandwich with a bag of chips and a soft drink—or a hefty fast food burger with extra cheese, a large order of French fries, and a "super-sized" soft drink. The afternoon hours feature an "energy-boosting" candy bar from a vending machine chased with another soft drink. Dinner is invariably a meat-and-potatoes affair with a white roll and margarine, some canned green beans for the health-conscious, followed by Neapolitan ice cream for dessert.

I figure by now that you already know this diet amounts to a prescription for poor health at best and disaster at worst. Virtually any departure from this typical American diet will make you feel better. There is very good reason that I refer to the standard American diet by its acronym—SAD!

The Vegetarian Diet

Vegetarian diets rank as perhaps the oldest of all specialty diets. Some people turn to vegetarian diets because of religious or philosophical beliefs, while others shun meats for fear of heart disease or to avoid the supposedly "bad" saturated fats found in animal foods.

Vegetarianism has the appearance of a great lifestyle. But there are different kinds of vegetarians. To clarify terminology, while all vegetarians avoid meat, fish, and fowl, lacto-ovo vegetarians add dairy and eggs, and lacto-vegetarians say yes to dairy but no to eggs. Vegans, who have risen tremendously in numbers during the last decade, generally consider themselves animal rights activists because they won't eat or use any animal products—no meat, no dairy, no honey, no leather, no silk, no cosmetics, and no soaps. Their motto is "never to eat or use anything that comes from something with a face." (The reason they don't eat honey is because honey is produced by bees.)

Variations of the vegetarian diet include the fruitarian diet (no definition needed).

Then there are the Hallelujah and Genesis diets, which are based on God's early instructions to Adam and Eve in the Garden of Eden to eat only grains, nuts, seeds, legumes, fruits, and vegetables (Genesis 1:29).

Summing up, pure vegetarianism plays into all the food phobias prevalent in our very phobic society. Furthermore, vegetarian apologists attribute virtually every problem of humanity to the consumption of meat, animal fat, and animal products.

Benefits

The chief benefit of the vegetarian diet is that the focus on fruits and veggies and avoidance of junk food decreases the toxic burden on the body. Vegetarianism is of tremendous value as a short-term cleansing diet.

Downside

The purist vegan diet is totally unsuitable for a long-term diet, however, because it deprives the body of essential nutrients available only from meat and animal products. These nutritional deficiencies are nothing to sneeze at and pose potentially deadly consequences to long-term health. Stephen Byrnes, Ph.D., N.D., the author of Diet & Heart Disease and Digestion Made Simple, published an in-depth article entitled "The Myths of Vegetarianism" in the Townsend Letter for Doctors and Patients. This article is the primary source for the following information about vegetarianism.

The goal of Dr. Byrnes was not to bash vegetarians but to correct the myth that vegetarianism is somehow a healthier way to live than going through life consuming meat or animal products, which vegans believe is a prescription for sickness and death. Proponents of vegetarianism justify this claim with a number of secondary myths that are widely cited but totally unsupported by scientific evidence. They include the following:

Myth: Meat consumption contributes to famine and depletes the earth's natural resources. The myth behind the myth is the simplistic idea that the solution to world hunger is for people to become vegetarians. Based on the claim that livestock dominate agricultural land that could be used to raise grains to feed the world's starving masses, the fact is two-thirds of the earth's landmass is unsuitable for farming but easily provides food for grazing animals.

To the charge that animals are fed grain that could be more efficiently used to feed the world's starving masses, Byrnes points out that two-thirds of the plants and plant products fed to animals are unsuitable for human consumption. Because animals and the plants are renewable resources, neither are in danger of depletion.

People do need to eat an abundance of plant products for good health, but the problem has never been a shortage of these foods. Rather, it's the equitable distribution as well as widespread poverty that's the complication. Even the Population Reference Bureau attributes the world hunger problem to poverty, not eating meat, and does not consider mass vegetarianism to be a solution to world hunger.

Myth: Vitamin B12—a nutrient that helps keep the body's nerve and blood cells healthy and helps make DNA, the genetic material in all cells— can be obtained from plant sources. This may be the most dangerous myth of all. Vegans who do not supplement their diets with vitamin B12 will eventually succumb to anemia—a potentially fatal condition. According to Byrnes, several studies indicate most, if not all vegans, have impaired B12 metabolism and low vitamin B12 concentrations.

Vegans simply do not get this vitamin from their diet because it can only be found in animal products like eggs, fish, red meat, and organ meats. Besides anemia, a deficiency in vitamin B12 can also cause fatigue and neurological disorders. Vitamin B12 is essential for cell division, energy, and the formation of red blood cells.

Many vegetarians believe they get vitamin B12 from eating tempeh (fermented soybean cake), spirulina (a type of algae), and brewer's yeast, but that's not really the case. Though these foods contain compounds called B12 analogs, these compounds cannot be metabolized by the body.

Some researchers believe that spirulina, although a generally healthy food, actually depletes vitamin B12 because the B12 analogs compete with vitamin B12 and inhibit the metabolism of the vitamin. Vitamin B12 is produced by fermenting bacteria in the large intestine, as vegans claim, but it must have "intrinsic factor" from the stomach to be absorbed, which makes this fermentation byproduct unusable by the body.

Thus, the only reliable sources for vitamin B12 are meat and fish and, to a lesser degree, dairy products.

Myth: Our needs for vitamin D can be met by sunlight. It's true that the body, in particular the skin, catalyzes the conversion of cholesterol into vitamin D, which manages calcium in bones and helps cells communicate properly. This conversion, however, only occurs in the presence of relatively rare UV-B rays, which are present only at certain times of the day, at certain latitudes, and at certain times of the year. Even then, depending on one's skin color, it would take as long as two full hours of continual sunning to get 200–400 IUs of vitamin D. Recent research indicates adults need even higher amounts of this vitamin.

And you can only soak up rays if there's sunlight. I was reminded of that when our family moved from the Sunshine State—Florida—to our Missouri ranchland in 2013. From Thanksgiving to Easter, we didn't see the sun very much, and when we did, those rays didn't feel very warm. Much of the northern half of the country has gray skies all winter long, so relying on sunlight is a fool's errand for at least half the year.

As for using supplementation, a limited number of plant foods contain a form of vitamin D called D2, but clinicians have reported disappointing results using D2 to treat conditions such as rickets, which are related to a vitamin D deficiency. Concerns about vitamin D deficiencies and rickets in vegetarians and vegans always exist because the full complex of this vital nutrient is only found in animal fats.

Myth: The body's needs for vitamin A can be entirely obtained from plant foods. This vitamin is all-important to the human diet because it allows the body to use proteins and minerals, enhances the immune system, fights infection, and ensures proper vision and reproduction. Unfortunately for vegetarians and vegans, the true form of vitamin A, or retinol, is found only in animal fats and organs such as the liver. The body can convert beta carotene from plants into vitamin A if bile salts are available, but bile secretion in the body is stimulated by the consumption of fat.

Even then, the conversion isn't very efficient. Butter and full-fat dairy foods from pastured cows are rich sources of vitamin A, as is cod liver oil.

Myth: Eating meat causes osteoporosis, kidney disease, heart disease, and cancer. This claim does not reconcile with historical fact and anthropological research, contrary to what you may have heard. All of the diseases mentioned became much more widespread in the 20th century, whereas people—and long-lived people at that—have been eating meat and animal fat for thousands of years. The truth is that recent studies demonstrate that vegan and vegetarian diets predispose women to osteoporosis because of the lack of protein from meat and calcium from dairy products.

As for kidney disease, meat contains complete proteins and vitamin D, both of which help maintain pH balance in the bloodstream. Meats that God has provided—beef, fish, and lamb—are good sources of magnesium and B6, which help limit the risk of kidney stones. Nothing in nutritional science supports the claim that eating meat causes cardiovascular problems. The French eat large amounts of meat with cream sauces and enjoy low rates of heart disease. The same is true in Greece.

The claim that eating meat causes cancer is based on a flawed study by Dr. Ernst Wynder in the 1970s, who said there was a link between animal fat intake and colon cancer. The "animal fats" turned out to be vegetable fats. Historically, studies of meat-eating peoples—including the people of the Bible—show they had very little incidence of cancer.

Myth: Saturated fats and dietary cholesterol cause heart disease, atherosclerosis, and/or cancer—and low-fat, low-cholesterol diets are healthier for people. This claim is rooted in the flawed "liquid lipids" hypothesis has been used to promote vegetarianism as the best insurance against heart disease.

The theory that saturated fats and cholesterol clog arteries has been effectively disproved by a number of highly respected scientists from many nations. Studies have shown that arterial plaque is primarily composed of unsaturated fats, particularly polyunsaturated ones, and not the saturated fat of animals, palm or coconut. The real culprit is trans fatty acids in such supposedly "healthy" foods as margarine, vegetable shortening, and foods made with them. A Swedish study confirmed previous findings linking vegetable oil intake with higher breast cancer rates.

The Framington Heart Study, often cited as "proof" of this myth, actually found that residents of Framington, Massachusetts, who ate more saturated fats, cholesterol, and calories had the lowest serum cholesterol levels! Vegetarian diets do not protect against heart disease or atherosclerosis. Recent studies have shown vegetarians to have higher homocysteine levels in their blood. (Homocysteine is a known cause of heart disease.)

Myth: Vegetarians live longer and have more energy and endurance than meat-eaters. One English vegetarian guidebook claimed that vegetarians "can expect to live nine years longer than meat-eaters." A witty commentator called this so-called life expansion "indulging in a bit of wishful thinking."

A comprehensive study of heart disease by Russell Smith, Ph.D., showed that death rates actually decreased as animal product consumption increased among some study groups. The longest-lived peoples on earth have all been meat-eaters, and the anthropological data from primitive societies do not support the contention that vegetarians live longer than meat-eaters.

Myth: Consumption of meat and saturated fat has increased in the twentieth century, with a corresponding increase in heart disease and cancer. The hard statistics say the opposite. Butter consumption dropped by more than two-thirds over the last century, but the incidence of heart disease and cancer skyrocketed. Explain that one. And while we're at it, beef consumption has risen, but meat-eating societies have lived virtually free of cancer and heart disease for centuries, so this cannot be a sole factor.

What has kept pace with the rise of heart disease and cancer is our consumption of trans-fatty acids, packaged foods, processed vegetable oils, carbohydrates, and refined sugar—items virtually unavailable to primitive societies of long-lived meat-eaters. I think you know where the blame should land.

Myth: Soy products are adequate substitutes for meat and dairy products. In Asia, soy products are never used as a primary food. They are used as condiments or side dishes in traditionally fermented forms. Unfermented soybeans and soy products are high in phytic acid, an anti-nutrient that carries minerals out of the body.

Vegetarians are known for their frequent mineral deficiencies; the high phytate content of grain and legume-based diets is to blame. Processed soy products are rich in trypsin inhibitors, which inhibit protein digestion. Some recent research indicates that soy's phytoestrogens (or isoflavones) could be causative factors in breast cancer, penile birth defects, infantile leukemia, and depressed thyroid function. They have caused infertility in every animal species studied so far as well.

Myth: The human body is not designed for meat consumption. Human physiology clearly refutes this false claim. The stomach's production of hydrochloric acid is unique to meat-eaters—and activates protein-splitting enzymes. This is not something found in herbivores.

Then there is the human pancreas, which produces a full range of digestive enzymes for handling both animal and vegetable foods. Our very physiology, including our dental structure, demonstrates we are "mixed feeders" or omnivores.

Myth: Animal products contain numerous harmful toxins. Dr. Byrnes comments, "If meat, fish, and eggs do indeed generate cancerous 'ptyloamines,' it is very strange that people have not been dying in droves from cancer for the past thousand years." It also seems strange to me that our Creator would recommend such foods in Leviticus and Deuteronomy, or that Jesus and the disciples would eat them, thereby validating them.

Commercially raised or farmed meat and animal sources may have some harmful contaminants in them (as do commercially farmed plant foods), but this can be avoided by consuming grass-fed organic meats, free-range eggs, and organic dairy products free of man-made chemical toxins.

Myth: Eating meat or animal products is less "spiritual" than eating only plant foods. I'm satisfied to know that Abraham prepared a calf for three angelic visitors. I'm glad to know that Isaac, Jacob, David, and Moses all ate meat, and Jesus partook of meat at the Last Supper, sharing fish with the disciples.

Most vegetarians are really "grain-etarians," "sugar-tarians," or "starch-etarians." The excessive consumption of carbohydrates can drive up insulin levels and jeopardize overall health. Health problems typically associated with vegetarianism include anemia, pallor, listlessness, and poor resistance to infection.

The Raw Food Vegan Diet

Raw food advocates never cook food before eating it, believing this weakens the potency of vitamins and minerals, destroys enzymes, and possibly introduces toxins. (One version of the raw food diet suggests eating raw meat as well as raw fruits and vegetables.)

Their premise is that cooking destroys food enzymes that help with digestion. By preserving these enzymes, we can digest food properly and assimilate nutrients.

Benefits

The raw food diet shares all the advantages of the vegetarian diet, which are earned by eating plenty of organic fruits, vegetables, and nuts—foods rich in the antioxidants (including vitamins C, E, and beta carotene) that prevent free radicals from damaging body tissue.

Downside

The raw food diet also shares all the drawbacks of the vegetarian diet. The raw food diet is notoriously lacking in quality protein, unless raw animal foods are included. This diet is very difficult to stay on and can be problematic with today's tainted food supply and lack of minerals, vitamins (most notably vitamins A, D, and B12), and essential fatty acids obtainable only from animal foods and/or animal fat.

Some raw food advocates supplement their raw vegetarian diet with raw animal products such as unpasteurized dairy products, raw eggs, uncooked meats, poultry, and fish. This combination offers many benefits, but they may be outweighed by the risk of raw food contamination due to parasites. In addition, some foods are easier to digest when cooked; people with gastrointestinal illnesses simply cannot tolerate a predominantly raw food diet.

Humans lack the enzyme cellulase, which is necessary for digesting plant fibers. In addition, undesirable intestinal microbes can ferment undigested sugar and fiber, which may produce gas, inflammation, and severe pain in certain individuals. I believe a healthy diet contains a combination of raw and cooked foods with plenty of raw foods. Those in seasonal climates will usually be better off consuming more cooked foods in the winter and more raw foods in the summer.

The Anti-*Candida* (Anti-Yeast) Diet

Many women are drawn to the anti-yeast diet because of chronic battles with *Candida* in the form of vaginal yeast infections and a myriad of other health problems often attributed to systemic *Candida* infections. *Candidiasis*, or chronic yeast overgrowth, is a disease caused by a yeast fungus, *Candida albicans*.

This yeast often breeds in the throat, mouth, digestive tract, and vaginal tract as well as on the skin. This same yeast, however, has valuable functions in the digestive tract as long as it's kept in check by other more beneficial microorganisms in the intestine. Once it grows out of control, this seemingly harmless yeast turns into an aggressive fungus that can cause serious intestinal problems and infections of the vagina, mouth, and throat. (The latter two are known as "thrush.")

In its most serious form, the Candida fungus grows into and through the walls of the intestine, allowing food particles, toxic waste, and yeast waste products to seep into the bloodstream. This serious condition is called leaky gut syndrome. Many cases of Candida occur after taking antibiotics that kill all bacteria in the gut. Candida microbes, resistant to antibiotics, remain active and take over when the friendly bacteria that would normally keep them in check die out.

Benefits

The anti-Candida diet is an attempt to starve the Candida fungus by elima
inating sugar in every form, including foods and beverages that contain sugar,
plus fresh fruit and fruit juices because Candida yeast feeds on sugars. Foods
fermented with vinegar such as soy sauce, beer, vinegar, sauerkraut, and pick-
les are also avoided as they may cause an exacerbation of the condition.

Naturally fermented foods using probiotic cultures are highly recommended in the fight against Candida. Avoiding these foods also lowers
carbohydrate consumption, which can help people balance blood sugar and
hormones and may also aid in weight management.

Downside

The standard medical community does not recognize candidiasis as a cona
dition. It may also be diagnosed much too often among alternative medicine
practitioners, who seem to readily blame yeast overgrowth for symptoms
when the root cause is the lack of balance in the gut flora and immune system
that keeps Candida albicans in check. Anti-Candida diets can be very diffia
cult to follow, and they exclude many healthy foods, including fruit and honey.

Following the Maker's Diet and adding probiotic supplements, especially
SBOs, are extremely effective against Candida and other fungi, working to
create a healthy balance of flora.

Balanced Macronutrient Ratios Diet ("the Zone")

The balanced macronutrient ratios diet advocates eating macronutrients
(carbohydrates, protein, and fat) in the ratio of 40 percent carbohydrate, 30
percent protein, and 30 percent fat. Promoters claim this diet will help you lose
weight, live longer, and lower the risk of heart disease.

Dr. Barry Sears, a biochemist, created the Zone diet, which he promoted in
his popular books while sounding the alarm about the danger of carbohydrate
overconsumption. His goal has been to produce a more balanced biochemical
state in the body by reducing carbohydrate intake to 40 percent while increasing protein intake to 30 percent. The Zone diet focuses on two blood-sugar
hormones—insulin (the fat-storing hormone) and glucagon (the fat-releasing
hormone)—and on a group of short-acting bioactive chemicals known as eicosanoids, which promote inflammation.

Balancing macronutrient ratios is a great improvement over the high-carb, low-fat diet. This philosophy leads to more balanced blood sugar levels, a reduction in inflammation, and weight loss as well.

Downside

The Zone diet fails to address the quality of the food you eat. There is also a noticeable shortage of the fat-soluble vitamins A and D in this diet. Dr. Sears strongly endorses soy protein isolates, which new research suggests can be highly allergenic and estrogenic; these isolates can be problematic for men and certain women as well. Soy is an inferior protein source containing high levels of phytic acid. (Exceptions are naturally fermented forms of soy.)

My recommendation? Follow the Maker's Diet, which is packed with super nutrition, healthy carbohydrate intake, and the highest quality protein and fat from sources such as organically raised meat, poultry, fish, eggs, and fermented dairy products. As we will discuss, this diet lowers insulin and inflammation levels naturally, thus reducing the levels of "bad" eicosanoids in the body, while also promoting healthy weight levels and reducing inflammation.

The Low-Carb Diet

When *The Maker's Diet* came out in 2004, the most popular diets were the low-carb diets. You remember them, right? They were diets like Dr. Atkins' New Diet Revolution, the South Beach Diet, Protein Power, and Sugar Busters.

The Atkins' Diet was the biggest and received the most publicity, although the South Beach Diet had its fans. Its popularity increased when medical studies acknowledged the diet's effectiveness as a weight-loss program.

All of these diets call for eating large amounts of protein and small amounts of carbohydrates—very small. What many people didn't know is that these low-carb diets essentially mimic fasting or starvation by reducing carbohydrate intake to a level that induces a physical state called ketosis, in which body metabolism speeds up and hunger urges are suppressed. Starved of glucose from carbohydrates, the body resorts to burning ketones, or the chemicals the body produces from fat. The keto diet, which aims to do this very thing, has become popular in the last couple of years with those looking for quick, dramatic weight loss and to improve their blood sugar levels.

Benefits

With the combination of hunger suppression, consuming fewer calories, and burning fat reserves, it must be stated that people on low-carb diets lose weight. Some promoters even claim that you can eat all the fat you want and still lose weight, which obviously sounds attractive. The body can tolerate the low-carb diet without substantial harm for certain periods of time. Under the supervision of a knowledgeable physician, a low-carb diet can be used to manage a host of illnesses, including obesity, GI disorders, childhood epilepsy, and certain types of brain tumors.

Downside

The popular versions of the low-carb diet cater to the current tastes and whims without discrimination about food choices. This makes low-carb diets really high-fat diets, not high-protein programs. The dietary suggestions for these regimens often make it very difficult to maintain a healthy ratio of omega-6 to omega-3 essential fatty acids.

Some of the recommended foods are terribly unhealthy, according to the biblical dietary guidelines as incorporated in the Maker's Diet. For instance, the late Dr. Robert C. Atkins suggested that dieters treat themselves to a heaping helping of pork rinds, calling them "the zero-carbohydrate consolation prize for corn or potato chip addicts." Bacon is another staple in low-carb diets, and many of the low-carb diets advocate the consumption of artificial sweeteners such as aspartame and sucralose, which may pose significant health risks.

The Food-Combining and Acid/Alkaline Diets

If Adam and Eve sat down in the garden for a hearty "food-combining" meal, you would see them carefully separate certain foods from others.

Many advocates believe that alkaline-forming foods are essential because humankind evolved from the alkaline environment of the ocean. Even aside from its non-biblical origins, the problem with the food-combining diet is that most of its suppositions are not based on scientific fact or historical evidence. No empirical evidence suggests that the body has trouble digesting certain foods when eaten in combination.

The acid-alkaline diet, which divides food into alkaline-forming and acid-forming foods, is the first cousin variation of the food-combining diet.

This type of diet sets a goal of eating 80 percent alkaline-forming foods and 20 percent acid-forming foods.

Benefits

Because most people tend to be overly acidic, both of these diets can be beneficial for those switching from a primarily junk-food diet. After learning about the food-combining diet years ago, I never eat melon with any other food, in accordance with food-combining adage that goes like this: "Melon—eat it alone or leave it alone."

Many people experience improved digestion by avoiding certain combinations of foods. If you notice certain food combinations are tough on your gut, it's best to avoid them. For the average person, however, most healthy foods eaten in combination are just fine and have been for thousands of years.

Downside

People on acid-alkaline and food-combining diets experience all the same challenges as those on vegetarian diets. Due to the lack of animal foods, they run the risk of long-term nutrient deficiencies.

The Blood Type Diet

I call the blood type diet an evolution-based diet because its promoters believe our food requirements "evolved" with mankind over 40 million years since prehistoric times in essentially four "flavors" that conveniently correspond with the body's blood types—O, A, B, or AB.

This is a diet philosophy popularized in the late 1990s by Peter D'Adamo, N.D., in his best-selling book Eat Right for Your Type. He maintains that modern people with type O blood are descended from the earliest humans, who were physically active and ate a diet composed mostly of the meat of large herbivorous mammals, but with little or no grain. Under such a scenario, I suppose it makes sense that today's "modern cavemen" with type O blood also require large amounts of meat and lots of exercise.

Type As descended from agrarian humans who were more docile, thrived on vegetables and fruit, and avoided meat and dairy products. Type Bs descended from nomadic herders and thrive on dairy products while requiring only moderate exercise. According to D'Adamo, Type ABs did not handle meat well, so they should eat fish, grains, and soy-based foods.

Proponents of the blood-type diet claim that lectins—or specialized proteins in foods such as cereals and beans—are incompatible with certain blood types, causing many ailments such as kidney failure, arthrosclerosis, and food allergies.

Benefits

The diet's virtues appear to be those of a low-calorie, healthy diet. For people who typically eat junk food, adopting the blood type diet will be an improvement, allowing them to take in fewer calories, exercise more, naturally lose weight, and feel better.

Downside

Aside from being unbiblical, this diet was viewed as a fad by the scientific community and many nutritionists in alternative circles back in its heyday. Its thesis remains unproven and without solid anthropological evidence.

New Age Programs

Once you depart from the solid foundation of biblical, historical, and common-sense nutrition, you enter the no-man's-land of New Age programs, unusual therapies, and odd diagnostic contraptions. Let the buyer beware!

You will find motivated and sincere people who claim each of these programs worked for them. I tried many of them during my desperate search for health, so I'm familiar with the territory, but nothing restored my health except the biblically grounded and scientifically proven foods of the Maker's Diet.

I know that desperate times require desperate measures, but before you commit to an alternative, looks-good-to-me diet from the bestseller list, take a chance on the historically correct and life-giving principles of the Maker's Diet. In the years since the original release of *The Maker's Diet*, I've been able to help thousands of others overcome serious health problems, turning their tragedy into triumph.

In the next chapter, you will meet several of these people who tell their dramatic success stories. Consider their seemingly hopeless health crises, and then share their surprise and joy in discovering the commonsense biblical diet that turned their lives around.

7

Seven Victims Find Victory

DISAPPOINTMENT IN MODERN MEDICINE IS THE HARD REALITY EXPERI-enced by millions of Americans. Some maintain they were lied to and even discarded by health-care systems and providers. Others simply exhausted all of their options in a search for health that was forever lost to disease, accidents, or nutrition-related health problems.

I wrote the previous paragraph more than ten years ago, before Barack Obama's spellbinding speech at the 2004 Democratic Party convention and before, of course, his election as the 44th president of the United States and the passage of his signature legislation, the Affordable Care Act. It's not my intention to stray into the political side of how our health-care system touches the lives of every American and every person living within our borders. But I do want to acknowledge this reality as I move forward in this chapter.

That said, while personal testimonies cannot take the place of scientifically controlled studies or independent research, neither should they be ignored or set aside. They are a vital part of the process of scientific inquiry and discovery.

This is why I have selected seven people who experienced significant results on the Maker's Diet. They represent a cross-section of people who first sought help through standard medical health care without success and were desperate enough to seek out a new approach to recover their health, as God intended them to enjoy. Some had been disappointed with the conventional and alternative medical community. Others received life-saving procedures but discovered that regaining their total health required more than was available from the conventional medical system.

Suffering the "System"

Let me affirm again that I understand that doctors, nurses, and other health-care providers, by and large, are sincere, highly gifted, and dedicated in their work. They are, however, part of a rapidly changing health-care system in this country that is becoming what some call an "unholy alliance" between the federal government, large insurance companies, the public health system, and the medical profession.

Each party brings its own agenda to the table, and some are motivated by goals that may not have the public's best interest at heart. Some for-profit health maintenance organizations (HMOs), for instance, have won nationwide disdain for their tendency to maximize profits while minimizing health-care services and expenditures to protect those profits, which is one of the reasons we saw the Affordable Care Act passed in 2010.

As the way of providing health care sorts itself out in Washington, far too often government bureaucrats and insurance underwriters, along with pharmaceutical companies, are influencing key medical treatment decisions, rather than the patients and their health-care providers. Other key decision makers avoid many proven alternatives, including virtually everything in the realm of proper nutrition and genuine health maintenance.

A Typical Scenario

The story is all too familiar, beginning with the long delays in crowded waiting rooms packed with sick people sneezing, coughing, and hacking uncontrollably. After being whisked into an antiseptic examination room, you wait another thirty minutes before seeing the doctor, who finally appears for a rushed ninety-second interview, which he uses to prescribe medications.

The result is predictable: you thank the doctor for his time, take your prescription script with you on the way out past the small receptionist window, and then you make the weary run to your friendly hometown pharmacist for the promised "cure in a bottle."

Add to that the ever-increasing problems of incorrect prescribing, over-prescribing of antibiotics, missed diagnoses, late diagnoses, and understaffed and underpaid hospital workers laboring in a fog of fatigue, often working in overcrowded conditions in buildings housing a host of deadly microbes, communicable diseases, and infectious staph infestations, well...taken together, you have a prescription for disaster! As my mother says, "The worst place for a sick person to be is in the hospital."

Each of the individuals introduced below came to me in desperation after every other medical promise had failed. Feeling helpless and almost hopeless, they agreed to try the Maker's Diet. The first testimonial is very special to me because it's from my grandmother, who died a couple of years after the original Maker's Diet was released. Grandma Rose, as I called her, was an amazing woman who overcame a lot in her long and rich lifetime.

~

GRANDMA ROSE

"Jordan, are you okay? Can I get you anything? Do you need your IV changed?"

The voice was very familiar to me. I heard those loving words night after night as I came in and out of delirium in the hospital—it was the concerned voice of Rose, my resilient, full-of-life Jewish grandmother.

This matriarchal champion stood by me in my battle to survive Crohn's disease, which I will never forget. Then, three years after my recovery, as I was enjoying life and planning my wedding, which was only three months away, Grandma Rose found herself in a life-and-death battle with cancer. According to her doctor, things weren't looking good.

Her cancer story began in the spring of 1999, when she began experiencing excruciating stomach pain and threw up constantly. Laboratory tests conducted in Florida, however, kept coming back normal. Her doctors wrote it off as a tough virus.

Grandma Rose traveled to Atlanta to visit my aunt and uncle but felt horrible and couldn't leave her guest room. She had to be lifted out of bed and helped in and out of the shower. Days turned into weeks of pain and nausea. My poor grandma had difficulty in keeping food down, the dry heaves, and excruciating abdominal pain.

The pain became so unbearable that Grandma fell into despair. She even asked my uncle to give her pills so she could "end it all." When he refused, she asked to be taken to the emergency room. Desperate to end the pain, she agreed to follow the gut instinct of a surgeon she had never met. He was certain something dangerous was going on that could only be found through exploratory surgery.

Facing the Facts

When my mother, Phyllis, heard that her mother was going to be cut open, she was furious. (Mom has a natural distrust of "knife-happy" surgeons, a feeling common to many in the natural health community.) But this time the doctor was right. When Grandma emerged from the anesthesia, the surgeon confirmed what she secretly suspected—she was dying from cancer.

He found multiple malignancies hidden beneath the larger internal organs, which explained why they had escaped detection. The malignancies included a goblet cell carcinoid in her appendix and stage IV ovarian cancer that had spread to her lymph nodes and portions of her small and large intestines. Ovarian cancer cells were also found in the pleural fluid, located in the cavity surrounding the lungs.

The experienced surgeon removed all of the cancer he found, cutting and taking away both ovaries, the appendix, some of the lymph nodes, and portions of the small and large intestines. But the ovarian malignancy was extremely advanced, and the cancer had spread to other sites.

Because Grandma Rose was in her late seventies and in a weakened state, chemotherapy and radiation were out of the question. The doctor told Rose she "needed to get her affairs in order" and had two years to live at most. Privately to our family, her doctor said she had six months to live—if that long.

I'll never forget the emotional phone call I received from Grandma Rose. "Jordan, you are my first grandchild," she said with a weak voice that quivered. "I want to live long enough to see you married. Maybe you can help me. Maybe you can find something for me." I had never heard Grandma sound so down before.

As we talked, I realized just how similar her trial was to my own. Her condition was extremely painful, and no one seemed to believe her description of the symptoms at first. She didn't know what was wrong, but now she did. The unrelenting suffering had stolen her hope—and her smile.

She had lost thirty pounds, felt terrible, and had lost her will to live—except for one thing. She really wanted to attend my upcoming wedding to my fiancée, Nicki, in Palm Beach Gardens just a few months away.

A Painful Challenge

Though the stakes were almost unbearable, I had no choice but to try to help my grandmother. All of her conventional medical options were exhausted.

I understood that I had to find a way to strengthen Grandma's immune system. She needed more than an increase in white blood cells and cytokines in her body—these components needed to be highly activated as well.

Tumor cells secrete "transforming growth factor-beta" (TGF-b), which renders immune cells inactive or ineffectual—even in large numbers. This factor also inhibits the proliferation of T-cells, reduces the cancer cell-killing power of tumor necrosis factor-alpha, and inhibits the ability of macrophages—our immune system's first line of defense—to destroy invaders. The result: the body believes its defense system is effectively attacking cancer cells when it isn't.

In addition to putting Grandma on the Maker's Diet, my research led me to particular polysaccharide peptides or glycoproteins that enhance macrophage and natural killer cell production and efficacy. They are found in greatest abundance in edible fungi and germinated grains and seeds. These compounds enhance production of cytokines, which facilitate cell-to-cell communication and optimize immune function. I had a hunch that these glyconutrients might overcome some of the deceptive methods of TGF-b.

Glyconutrient compounds were abundant in most primitive diets, but they are virtually absent from modern Western diets heavy in refined foods. Edible mushrooms are the richest source of these compounds (the healing powers of mushrooms have been known for more than five thousand years). Positive research findings on the medicinal powers of mushrooms became prominent in research literature in the 1980s.

Several varieties—but not including the popular button mushroom from the grocery store—offer immunomodulatory, lipid-lowering, anti-tumor, and other beneficial or therapeutic health effects without any significant toxicity. These benefits are so promising that some of the most potent anti-cancer drugs under development by pharmaceutical scientists are based on the glyconutrient compounds found in these mushrooms. I was able to obtain various mushroom preparations containing carefully studied varieties and provide them to Grandma Rose.

Her body was able to utilize all of the "body ready" phytochemicals and phytonutrients available in the mushrooms, which she combined with the Maker's Diet immediately following her surgery.

The results were an amazing success.

A Rose Blooming Again!

Not only did Grandma Rose gain back much of her lost weight, but her energy and physical appearance improved to the point where she told us that hadn't felt this good in thirty years. Her digestion made a dramatic improvement.

And then came the stunning news after her first round of CAT scans following her surgery: Grandma Rose was cancer free! Even the fatty liver that she developed was gone.

Not only was Grandma Rose at my wedding, but she loved getting on the dance floor with me for a special dance in front of the entire wedding party and our invited guests. She and I did the foxtrot to a song that I sung and recorded just for her—"Just the Way You Look Tonight," made famous by one of Grandma's favorite singers, Frank Sinatra. Within my family, there were a lot of moist eyes because we knew how special this moment was to my grandmother.

Grandma Rose continued to be the picture of health following the wedding. On Labor Day 2001, Grandma Rose described her victorious battle before the Cancer Control Society's twenty-sixth annual convention in Universal City, California. "Four years after the discovery of my cancer, my CAT scans show no evidence of cancer. My energy levels are that of a twenty-year-old. With help from my grandson, I hope to see my great-grandchildren grow up."

She didn't get her wish. After a couple of years, she grew complacent about her near-miss from death and abandoned the Maker's Diet for sugary treats like doughnuts and vanilla ice cream. Then the cancer came back, and Grandma Rose was all ears again. Nicki was pregnant with our first son, Joshua, so she wanted desperately to see him. We all thought she was making great strides until the time she fell down our staircase during a visit, badly bruising her head and shattering her elbow on our marble floor.

During her recovery, the cancer became a death grip that Grandma Rose couldn't shake. She died before Joshua was born, and I mourned the loss of a special woman who meant more to me than she would ever know.

But there are happier stories to include in this chapter, which starts with Bob, who was dealing with a cancer diagnosis of his own.

≈

BOB'S STORY

I was devastated when I was given the life-changing news that I had stage III lymphoma cancer. Immediately, I started researching the available treatments and diet changes that would give me the best chance for a quality life and help me live the longest possible amount of time.

After consulting with my doctor and praying about what God wanted me to do, I chose to go with chemotherapy. After receiving five treatments, my hair fell out, and I was fighting nausea and fatigue.

When my son called to tell me that he had read about Jordan Rubin's incredible story and his health program called the Maker's Diet, I knew I had to meet Jordan. When I contacted him, he was unbelievably gracious and said I could call him. I immediately did so, and when we talked on the phone, I was so taken with his knowledge about good health that I boldly asked Jordan if I could jump on a plane and meet him in West Palm Beach. He said yes, and when we saw each for the first time, he went through the Maker's Diet with me. After my visit, I decided to continue chemotherapy while following the Maker's Diet and food supplement program very diligently.

My oncologist warned me that after my next series of treatments for stage III lymphoma cancer I would feel extremely weak and nauseated—much more than the initial five treatments. He also insisted that I go on disability because my energy level and blood count would drastically drop in the next few weeks.

Nonetheless, I began the Maker's Diet, including the food supplements recommended to me. I also followed Jordan's suggestion to observe a seven-day juice fast to detoxify and cleanse my system. I was sixty-five pounds overweight and had little energy to do anything else at the time.

A week in, I took my next chemotherapy treatment and waited for my energy level to hit rock bottom, as my doctor predicted. To my delight and great surprise, the nausea and fatigue were almost nonexistent! According to the doctor, my blood counts never dropped. What a difference the diet change and food supplements made.

The nurses at the doctor's office asked how I was, and when I told them how good I was feeling, they couldn't believe it! I mentioned that I was doing this program called the Maker's Diet, which they noted on my chart.

A few weeks later, I received the toughest chemotherapy treatment yet (five separate drugs), and the results were the same—very little side effects. This chemotherapy session happened just two days before Christmas when my son and his family flew in to visit with us. Would you believe that we had nine people in the house for one week and that I did the grocery shopping for every-one, cooked most of the meals, and entertained four grandchildren all under five years of age? Where did I get the energy I wasn't supposed to have? I am convinced I owe it to the Maker's Diet.

After New Year's, I stopped the program for about three days, just to see how I would do. Without receiving the nutrients from the Maker's Diet, I found myself extremely weak and hardly able to get up off the couch. I imme-diately started back on the program again and regained my strength the next day! That convinced me more than ever that the Maker's Diet was making a huge difference in my health.

In mid-January, my cancer was restaged by CAT and PET scans. The doctor, who is normally very low key, came bouncing energetically into the examina-tion room and shouted, "This is incredible. In my fifteen years of practice, this is the best lymphoma scan report I have ever seen. The lymph nodes have shrunk back to normal, and there is no sign of cancer anywhere!"

My wife and I were overcome with joy and excitement at the awesome report and answer to so many prayers. Not only did I progress better than anyone expected, but I lost twenty-five pounds and felt better than I had in years.

~

DOUG'S STORY

My journey began when I decided to make one last-ditch desperate attempt to correct a deteriorating physical condition that had plagued me for five long years.

It all began when I started experiencing recurring symptoms of heart-burn that rapidly progressed into a chronic acid reflux condition. I was unable to digest my food—regardless of what I ate—without bringing it back up repeatedly.

This took place over and over for forty-five minutes to an hour after each meal. This painful condition began to wreak havoc on me physically, emotionally, and socially. My eating habits became increasingly erratic. I often ate in seclusion to avoid any embarrassment associated with this condition, which I later learned was called GERD (gastroesophageal reflux disease).

I did some research and learned that GERD was a generic term applied to any common acid reflux or heartburn condition. I also learned that my particular case of GERD was anything but common when I visited my doctor seeking a diagnosis and a conventional medical remedy. That doctor's visit began an eighteen-month barrage of seemingly endless paperwork and referrals as I bounced from one specialist to the next within my HMO health insurance plan.

After running a number of diagnostic procedures (upper GI series, upper endoscopy, stomach-emptying study, manometry tests, etc.), my gastroenterologist declared that I had a severe case of GERD. There were also complications noted in my report: a gaping hiatal hernia; a duodenal ulcer; and an abnormally slow-emptying stomach, which emptied at a rate 75 percent slower than normal for a male my age. My prognosis wasn't good.

These complications, combined with the substantial reflux I was experiencing, made it very difficult to treat my GERD symptoms. It seemed that each health practitioner I sought for medical advice told me that GERD symptoms as complex and severe as mine were the leading cause of esophageal cancer. Hearing the word cancer got my attention. I was ready to exhaust every effort to combat my health problems.

I began a three-year search during which I tried three conventional prescription remedies, two mail-order prescriptions from Canada (not approved yet in the U.S.), and one prescription from Europe. Each "remedy" provided a host of side effects such as constant nausea, sleeplessness, and headaches—but none of them alleviated the reflux.

My desperation and hopelessness grew with each futile attempt at a cure. Finally, a specialist at the University of Miami Hospital told me my last remaining option was an uncommon surgical procedure called a Laparoscopic Nissen. The surgery would require the removal of the upper third of my stomach so it could be tied around the bottom of my esophagus. This sounded like a fate worse than death.

I avoided this grisly procedure by ignoring my problem for the next two years, even though there was a constant burning sensation in my throat and haunting fear of life-threatening throat cancer. When I could no longer stand the awful way I felt, I contacted my specialist again, who pleaded with me to undergo the Laparoscopic Nissen surgery. That was my only solution, he said.

Feeling like I had to cave in, I reluctantly scheduled a preoperative appointment with the hospital.

On the very same day that I scheduled my preoperative appointment, fate took a lucky turn. I just "happened" to share the details of my circumstances with a co-worker whom I really didn't know. That conversation became a life-altering moment. The guy's next sentence was, "Have you ever heard of Jordan Rubin?"

I said no without showing a shred of interest, but my co-worker was so persistent that he persuaded me to look at Jordan's website. That's when I was introduced to Jordan's amazing chronicle of his life-and-death battle with Crohn's disease. I felt a newfound inspiration budding inside me. I sensed this could be my last opportunity to avoid being butchered like a barnyard pig.

What happened next was nothing short of miraculous. I excitedly called the contact number on the website, and the customer service representative on the other end sounded strangely familiar. He turned out to be an old friend and co-worker of mine who was also a childhood friend of Jordan Rubin. He arranged for me to talk with this health expert.

Jordan's confidence impressed me immediately. I distinctly remember the kind and determined look in his eyes as I described my symptoms and mentioned that I had already booked a preoperative appointment for esophageal surgery. His confidence radiated from what he had overcome personally, and he had an absolute belief in the Maker's Diet. At the end of our meeting, he said, "If you're willing, I think I can help." The reassuring way he made this simple statement gave me a sense of optimism and hope I hadn't felt since my troubles began.

Jordan familiarized me with the Maker's Diet, recommending a dietary program and certain nutritional supplements, going to great lengths to describe the synergistic effect his program would have on my prevailing symptoms and on my overall health as well.

This was extremely exciting to me because for months I had been experiencing a number of other symptoms that alarmed me. I was almost embarrassed to discuss these symptoms with Jordan, fearing he would consider me to be some kind of hypochondriac. Yet, I felt I needed to make the most of this unique opportunity.

I went on to describe the strange malaise spells I'd get every three to four weeks. Lasting two or three days, these achy, bone-tired lethargic feelings rendered me almost nonfunctional.

Jordan empathized with everything I described to him because he had been down that horrible digestive tract road himself—and had emerged triumphant. Our conversation that day marked a turning point for me. I knew I was set on the right path, and I fervently began the Maker's Diet. I was unwaveringly determined to finally restore the most vital asset I possessed—my health.

The day I began the Maker's Diet was the last day I ever experienced GERD! I can still hardly believe it's true. I haven't had one iota of regurgitation from the very first dose of a digestive enzyme.

The protocol Jordan put me on included a digestive enzyme, a probiotic, a mushroom blend, an anti-inflammatory, a water purifier, an acid-relief formula, a super green food, cod liver oil, and lastly (yet most importantly) my strict adherence to the Maker's Diet.

Today I have absolutely no sign of the GERD or any of the related heartburn symptoms, and my energy levels have remained high with each passing day.

There's really no way to appropriately thank someone who gave me my life back…and I don't exaggerate when I say that. It's my prayer that many of you who are suffering from acid reflux and GERD symptoms will read my story and hold on to the hope that your prayers can be answered as well.

CHRISTIAN'S STORY

It was a cool Florida winter day, with a temperature of 65 degrees, slightly overcast skies, and strong prevailing winds when the course of my life was altered forever. And there I was, lying on the ground in agonizing pain. *This can't be happening!* I thought to myself.

Only split seconds earlier, while on patrol as a security guard for a luxury community, I was struck by a rather large SUV. The incident happened at lightning speed, but the moment seemed to last for an eternity.

Life throws a curve ball once in a while, and this was a doozy. At the time, I was on top of the world. I had just ended my service with the United States Air Force and was looking forward to serving the community as a deputy sheriff in West Palm Beach. Even more exciting at the time, my amateur boxing career was on the verge of exploding.

After the accident, though, my self-esteem hit a downward spiral. I found comfort in a lot of things—but my favorite was food. Because I could no longer train—and couldn't get out of bed for weeks—I had plenty of time to get well acquainted with two very good friends of mine—Ben & Jerry...the ice cream. As time went on, so did the pounds. I ballooned from a muscular six-foot, 200-pound hard-body physique to a marshmallow body shape weighing in at 270 pounds. I didn't even recognize the person I saw in the mirror.

The more depressed I felt, the more I ate. What a vicious cycle! I didn't know what to do. I kept my natural defense mechanism on the alert for any fat jokes that came my way so I could beat people to the punch line and make the joke on myself. That was the way I handled the feeling of rejection from all of my fit and thin friends.

I tried other ways to lose weight, but as a former athlete, the only effective method I had ever known was working out. But two herniated disks in my lower back and a bum left knee, along with the additional weight gain, removed the exercise option. It didn't help matters that problems with my insurance prevented me from getting the surgery I desperately needed.

So I had a decision to make: Would I keep living in this overweight, achy, tired, and depressed body? Or would I take back the control of my health I had forfeited and decide to do something about it?

I was introduced to a health program called the Maker's Diet shortly thereafter. At first, I dismissed it as just another diet, a fad one at that, but I couldn't get it out of my mind. Fed up with my predicament and facing my upcoming wedding, the choice was simple. I don't believe in coincidences, which is why I believe God gave me the unique opportunity to follow the Maker's Diet.

Just from the name I knew that God was in complete control and had heard my cries for help. This diet may be your answer as well. There are no coincidences in life, right?

I saw results immediately. Losing five pounds my first week was exciting and bolstered my faith in the path I was on. The funny thing was that I thought that being on a diet meant limiting the amount of food I was eating. With the Maker's Diet, though, I felt as if I was eating more than I ever had before.

After the second week, people started noticing and commenting on how good I was looking. Trust me, with my low self-esteem, I was sopping it up like a sponge in water.

The weight kept pouring off as I adhered to the diet and nutritional supplements, but my health wasn't the only thing that was improving. My self-worth was increasing as well. I woke up excited about life again, and I wasn't afraid to walk in front of the mirror without my shirt on. My knee and back pain decreased over a period of time, and my energy level skyrocketed from where it was before.

After twelve weeks, I had dropped forty pounds and was down to 230 pounds. Another fantastic result was that my back pain and knee pain improved to the point where I was able to get back in the gym and play pick-up basketball games.

Simple Conclusion

One by one, desperate people just like Rose, Bob, Doug, and Christian contacted me for help. While I do not consider myself a miracle worker, I do have great confidence in the Great Physician, who heals all our diseases (Psalm 103:3). Nothing matches His wisdom concerning His creation, including the ideal human diet and natural treatments for our most common ailments.

Before you examine the nuts and bolts of the Maker's Diet in the next chapter, I wanted you to consider the diet plan's effect on these people who were desperate for any glimmer of hope in their health situation—including my grandmother, who prayed for just a few more months of life so that she could see me get married. They represent a great number of people who enjoy restored health today as a result of making the decision to try the Maker's Diet.

There are more than two million copies of the Maker's Diet in print, so it's highly conceivable that millions have tried my health plan based upon the

Bible. Three of those persons were on the staff of the church I was attending when the original book was released. At the time, I asked them to share their stories, which they were glad to do.

I want to end this chapter with their before-and-after stories:

≈

JOANN'S STORY

Before: I guess I was sick and tired of being sick and tired. I think that pretty well sums up my attitude at the time. I've always had minor health problems all my life, so I got used to them. As you get older, though, those aches and pains become more noticeable.

Throughout my married life, all thirty years, my husband had his share "in sickness" and very little "in health" when it came to his life partner. I can't say I had major health issues, but they were enough for him to greet me each morning with this question: "How are you feeling today?"

I appreciated his love and concern, and I knew his question was sincere. He even measured the pause between the time he asked the question and the time it took me to answer to gauge my health. So after starting the Maker's Diet 40-Day Health Experience, my number-one goal was to feel so wonderful that my husband's first question every day wouldn't be, "How are you feeling today?"

I had other goals as well: not waking up in the middle of the night with a headache; seeing my blood pressure stabilize throughout the month; saying goodbye to my migraines; and for my hair to quit falling out.

After: I am still in shock. I never thought I'd feel so wonderful inside and out. I never thought I'd feel younger and more alive. I never thought I'd find myself smiling more.

As for my other goals:

1. I didn't want to wake up in the middle of the night with a headache; the headaches stopped.
2. I wanted my blood pressure to stabilize; throughout the forty days, I had one elevation, and it was not even "that time" of the month. (Speaking of my menstrual cycle, I had no BP

elevations or mood swings, and it was a lighter, more normal flow.)

3. I wanted my migraines to go away; I did not have one migraine the whole forty days!

4. I wanted my hair to quit falling out; my hair still fell out, but that's from the blood pressure medication I took many years ago. I knew my hair would not stop falling out overnight.

Another thing in the back of my mind was what these forty days would do for my husband…or our marriage. My husband needed to lose weight, so when he saw the effort I was putting in, he joined me on the Maker's Diet.

My heart melted when he came home from work one night and announced, "I feel great!" He lost a significant amount of weight, and to keep losing, he eagerly exercised and was careful to eat correctly. He was not tempted by candies or goodies at work. I'm so proud and pleased for him. But I also think the Lord softened his heart to be open to this opportunity.

And the grand prize happened when we were invited to an anniversary ball at our local Elk's club. I fit into the evening gown I wore to our daughter's wedding rehearsal dinner years ago, and my husband wore the same white dinner jacket and tuxedo pants. I cannot remember my husband ever looking so handsome—nothing too tight, nothing uncomfortable.

Then something wonderful happened. He looked at me and said, "You're looking real sexy!" And I felt it. I was so happy inside and out.

Hearing my husband say, "You're looking real sexy!" sure outclasses "How are you feeling today?"

≈

CAROLYN'S STORY

Before: At one time, I became very ill with mononucleosis, which I never seemed to recover from. I spent months at a time taking antibiotics and penicillin. I eventually had a tonsillectomy done and saw some improvement, but never complete healing. I suffered from fatigue on a daily basis. I never woke up refreshed and found it difficult to get through the day without enough energy. I also got sick very easily; if I was around someone who was ill, I was sure to get what they have.

I was diagnosed as having IBS (irritable bowel syndrome) and suffered from severe bloating, constipation, irregular bowel movements, distension, and cramping. This was a chronic, difficult thing to deal with over the years.

Before going on the Maker's Diet, I was engaged in a regimented exercise and eating routine with a personal trainer, which produced excellent results for a time. I toned up and ate only low-sodium and low-sugar foods. I was feeling well physically and had more energy during the day, but I knew it wasn't a program that would heal my body over the long term. I also didn't like how the food choices were extremely limited. No wonder I lost the drive to stay in that program.

Unfortunately, I got so busy with my job and master's degree course load that I neglected my health greatly. I doubled my dress size, going from a size 6 or 8 to a size 12 or 14.

I looked forward to the forty days as a time set aside to concentrate on healing and learning how to eat well. I specifically targeted my physical health, hoping to both lose weight and cleanse my bowels of any disease.

After: I cannot say enough about my journey through the Maker's Diet 40-Day Health Experience. I was challenged and blessed beyond measure by my involvement and witnessed critical changes in my overall health, which I had been praying for desperately over the years.

I finally got some answers about what foods I needed to avoid for optimal health. It was amazing how getting educated about proper nutrition—removing toxins, hormone-enhanced, chemically altered food, and introducing food in its natural form as our Maker created it—can change one's complete perspective about eating and enhance well-being.

For the first time in my life, I recognized how my body actually responded to foods not on the Maker's Diet. I had three difficult days where I ate foods off the diet, and each day I really felt the negative results of those choices within hours. My stomach cramped up and became distended. I got headaches and felt foggy and fatigued. It is almost like these foods were toxic to my body; my body wanted to repel them immediately.

I'm now certain that I was allergic to particular foods I had been eating on a frequent basis before starting this diet. My body just couldn't process them.

Typically, I would require a nap on both Saturday and Sunday afternoons to get myself ready physically for another week of labor. I can honestly tell you that I only took one nap while I was on the whole diet! There were some days when I thought, I should lie down and rest, only to find that I was not tired! This was truly amazing for me.

Being on the Maker's Diet made me far more productive at work as well. I have an intense job researching and writing all day, but now I can concentrate better, process more quickly, and be more efficient.

Much of the reason I have more energy is that my sleep has been more restful. My gut and my brain are working together! The three or so times I ate food off the diet, I didn't sleep nearly as well…so there is definitely a connection.

I'm sure my bowels were cleansed as well, which was a huge prayer concern for me. I believe with all my heart that the Maker's Diet helped my body learn how to absorb good bacteria and expel bad bacteria.

I also found that my skin became very clear and clean. This was the biggest area that I have gotten comments from others. They noticed a glow in my skin and a reduction in tiny lines around my eyes. I attributed this to removing chemicals, hormones, and pesticides from my foods and from following Jordan's recommendations for clean hygiene.

Since I got healthier, I have not missed one single opportunity to use the hygiene system, which changed my life. Here's an example: in the past, I have always gotten sick from flying on a plane. I can remember going on two round-trip flights while on the Maker's Diet, and I didn't have a sniffle—let alone the ear infections and bronchial infections I typically experience.

It was wonderful to do this diet with my boyfriend. We prayed about targeting particular areas such as diet before we committed in marriage, and guess what—it worked! We have supported one another, gotten educated together, and cooked together. We spent a lot more time at home because this diet simplified our life perspective, which was invaluable for us. Before we married, he said, "We're starting a legacy of health for our family." And we have.

I'm excited to work with him as one to build a family on God's wisdom and provisions. Proverbs 24:3–4 says, "Through wisdom a house is built, and by understanding it is established; by knowledge the rooms are filled with all precious and pleasant treasures." God has provided us with this wisdom through the Maker's Diet.

There's so much to say about how the Maker's Diet impacted me. I'm so thankful for the opportunity I had to take part in the Maker's Diet, which changed my life forever.

~

KIM'S STORY

Before: My incentive to get serious about my weight problem began when I started the Maker's Diet. At the time, I was at my heaviest weight ever.

Sure, I was active in high school and college, but after hitting my mid-thirties, it was harder to stay in shape, even though I was a children's pastor and keeping up with kids, but that was just on Sunday mornings. On the eating side, I didn't snack a lot, and I drank lots of water. I usually ate two big meals a day, skipping breakfast. I guess you could say my life was stressful. I moved to South Florida from Tennessee a few years ago not knowing anyone, so there were some adjustments to be made.

Grappling with all the adjustments had an effect on my mental and emotional health, which I believe has affected my physical health. I do see how stress affects your weight. The only thing I felt like I had going for me was my spiritual health, which the enemy tried to use against me during difficult times.

I didn't feel good about my appearance and had learned to hide my weight very well. Plus, I was constantly tired and usually had to push myself to work out.

Nonetheless, I committed myself to the forty days of the Maker's Diet. My goal was that this health plan would jump-start my metabolism, give me more energy, and change my lifestyle of eating habits. I didn't want this to be a forty-day fad and then go back to the "good ol' days."

I was ready to start feeling good about myself again and having a body—a temple—to reflect a healthy image. I desired balance in the areas of physical, mental, spiritual, and emotional health.

After: Wow! What an unbelievable forty days! Words can only briefly touch on how I feel. As stated in my "before" essay, I was not liking the way my body looked, and that affected many areas in my life. But I can definitely say today that I feel like a new person. I totally committed to this plan and faithfully worked out three times a week. I saw and felt a significant difference.

My overall attitude became healthier as well. I was determined to stick with the Maker's Diet even through the detox and occasional cravings for "bad" foods weren't easy. I gave up all caffeine and drank only water. I ate the foods that were recommended and came up with some new recipes. I didn't have to spend much time thinking about the foods to eat and preparing them during the forty-day health experience.

Living the Maker's Diet became part of my daily ritual—a habit. My whole being—spiritual, mental, physical, and emotional—became healthier and happier. The result was an in-shape Kim that I used to know years ago.

≈

8

Return to the Maker's Diet

THE SIMPLE REASON THE MAKER'S DIET CAN POSITIVELY AFFECT SO many different health problems is that it improves the health of the entire body, especially the digestive tract, which affects virtually all other bodily systems. The healing of the digestive system, in turn, positively affects the immune system, endocrine system, heart, lungs, blood supply, brain, and total nervous system. This proven health protocol involves a conscious return to the proteins, fats, carbohydrates, and additional micronutrients originally provided by our Creator for His highest creation—mankind.

As I discuss the basis of the Maker's Diet in this chapter, I first want to refute several popular myths about the basic food groups. To the uninitiated, let me warn you—you may be *shocked*. Much of the information you are about to read has been confirmed by numerous double-blind, placebo-controlled, scientific studies conducted over many years as well as by thousands of years of history. Rest assured, you have not read this information in the mainstream magazines, books, and television programs that are supposedly leading us to better health.

Understanding Our Roots

Just one hundred and fifty years ago, the diet of the average American was dramatically different from our SAD (standard American diet) table fare today. Widespread "mono-agriculture," with a concentration on single-crop farmlands using chemical fertilizers and pesticides, was unheard of back then, so the typical diet consisted mostly of meat from wild animals; fish caught from lakes, streams, and oceans; wild grain and seeds; raw, unpasteurized dairy products; and fruits and vegetables from the local farmer. (Of course, the menu varied significantly, depending on where you lived and the time of the year.)

Because the Creator made us with a perpetual pattern in mind, it shouldn't surprise you to learn that you crave the same foods, in their natural state, that your ancestors consumed. Our physical bodies were engineered as marvelous, highly tuned machines, genetically set for nutritional requirements established from the beginning of time.

Human physiology and biochemistry are geared for the foods the Creator intended for us to eat, not for the high-speed output of frozen dinners coming off the assembly line or bags of burgers and fries handed out by fast-food restaurants. (By my estimate, more than half of the "foods" commonly consumed today—like bacon-topped hamburgers or garlic fries—were not eaten by our ancestors.)

Our ancestors consumed 30 to 65 percent of their daily calories (and up to 100 grams of fiber a day) from a wide variety of fresh fruits and vegetables. That is why, long before the discovery of vitamins, people who had access to healthy foods lived extremely long lives without vitamin deficiencies or major illnesses. Their protein needs were met by consuming pasture-fed animals, wild game, and fish that were rich in highly beneficial omega-3 fatty acids and CLA (conjugated linoleic acid). These fats protected our ancestors against diseases such as cancer, diabetes, and heart disease.

The Maker's Proteins

The word *protein* is derived from the Greek word *proteus*, which literally means of primary importance. *Proteus* is translated into Latin as "primaries," meaning that it's the primary constituent of the body. The human body requires twenty-two amino acids to build body organs, muscles, and nerves, as well as and much more. Our physiology gives us the capacity to convert amino acids into proteins that combat invading protozoa, bacteria, and viruses. Altogether, your body builds or uses around fifty thousand different proteins, including five thousand specialized proteins called enzymes.

Under normal conditions, the healthy human body can manufacture all but eight of the twenty-two amino acids from healthy food sources entering the body. This means that these eight essential amino acids must come from other sources outside the body. If even one of these eight essential amino acids is missing, the body is unable to synthesize the other proteins it needs—no matter how much protein you eat.

Vegans and vegetarians won't like hearing this, but animal protein is our only complete protein source, providing all eight essential amino acids. When your body fails to get the essential amino acids and protein it needs, you begin to lose myocardial (heart) muscle, which may contribute to coronary heart disease.

Properly prepared (germinated or fermented) seeds, legumes, and cereal grains represent the best sources of protein in the vegetable kingdom, but they—along with all other plant foods—are low in three important amino acids: tryptophan, cystine, and threonine. Other sources are low in additional protein components, which is why many vegetarians emphasize eating from a variety of vegetable sources.

Popular protein powders, which are actually protein isolates, are derived from soy, egg whites, whey, and casein in a manufacturing process that uses high temperatures or harsh chemical additives that leave the protein virtually useless. Studies show that soy protein isolates in such powders tend to be high in mineral-blocking phytates, thyroid-depressing phytoestrogens, and potent enzyme inhibitors that depress growth and may even cause cancer.

The three key essential amino acids crucial to the health of the brain and nervous system are methionine, cysteine, and cystine, which are abundant in eggs and meat. While the consumption of organic fruits and vegetables is an obvious and important foundation of the Maker's Diet, the human body cannot function optimally without certain proteins and fats available only from animal sources. Just so you know, the Maker's proteins are rarely if ever supplied by man's mass production techniques.

Animal meats and dairy products purchased from grocery stores are prone to contamination from pesticides, herbicides, and chemical fertilizers as well as the common overuse of antibiotics and growth hormones in large-scale commercial feedlots, making these food sources downright dangerous.

For these and other reasons, I recommend only animal proteins from beef, lamb, goat, buffalo, venison, elk, and other clean red meats; fish with fins and scales from oceans and rivers; chicken, turkey, and other poultry organically raised in a free-range setting. I also recommend meats harvested from wild sources, which are becoming more widely available in your grocery store or local health food store.

Under no circumstances do I recommend pork or pork products, shellfish, or any of the other biblically unclean meats such as the ostrich and emu as sources of protein.

The Maker's Fats

As I have mentioned throughout this book, the Bible gives incredible information on health, especially diet. The foods eaten by the Israelites made them the healthiest people on the planet during ancient times. In reading the dietary instructions of the Bible, I wouldn't blame many health-conscious people for asking the same question: How could the Creator claim that fats are healthy food sources for human beings? Doesn't He know that saturated fats and cholesterol are the main causes of heart disease and cancer?

Contrary to something I refer to as the "cholesterol myth" that links saturated fat and dietary cholesterol with coronary heart disease, many saturated fats are actually good for you. This truth may not be easy to believe, but it is still true, nevertheless.

Dr. Michael DeBakey, the famous heart surgeon who died in 2008, studied 1,700 patients with hardening of the arteries and found no relationship between the level of cholesterol in the blood and the incidence of atherosclerosis. The Medical Research Council found that men eating butter—a key biblical fat—ran half the risk of developing heart disease as those eating margarine, a man-made fat that is often indigestible and toxic. A study comparing Yemenite Jews in Israel who ate butter against those consuming margarine and vegetable oils yielded similar results.

Saturated fats are not the "dietary demons" behind modern diseases. The truth—as revealed by the teaching in the Bible, anthropological evidence from past civilizations, and recent scientific research—makes it clear that saturated fats play a crucial role in body chemistry.

A list of the key roles of saturated fats is found in Nourishing Traditions, co-authored by Sally Fallon, a renowned nutritional researcher, and Mary Enig, Ph.D., an international expert in the field of lipid (fat) biochemistry:

* Saturated fatty acids constitute at least 50 percent of all cell membranes.

* At least 50 percent of dietary fat we consume should be saturated, otherwise calcium cannot be effectively incorporated into the skeletal structure.
* Saturated fats actually lower Lp (a), a key substance in the blood that indicates proneness to heart disease.
* Saturated fats protect the liver from alcohol and other toxins, such as those contained in nonsteroidal anti-inflammatory drugs (NSAIDs).
* Saturated fats enhance the immune system.
* Without saturated fats, we cannot properly utilize essential fatty acids such as the all-important omega-3 fatty acids.
* Saturated 18-carbon stearic acid and 16-carbon palmitic acid provide the preferred fuel for the heart, which is why the fat around the heart muscle is highly saturated.
* Short- and medium-chain saturated fatty acids found in butter, coconut, and palm oil have important antimicrobial properties. They protect us against harmful microorganisms in the digestive tract.

The authors summarize their study with this astounding statement: "The scientific evidence, honestly evaluated, does not support the assertion that 'artery-clogging' saturated fats cause heart disease. Actually, evaluation of the fat found in clogged arteries reveals that only about 26 percent is saturated. The rest is unsaturated, of which more than half is polyunsaturated."

The author of the study cited by Fallon and Enig—Uffe Ravnskov, M.D., Ph.D.—wrote this:

Studies of African tribes have shown that intakes of enormous amounts of animal fat [do] not necessarily raise blood cholesterol; on the contrary it may be very low. Samburu people, for instance, eat about a pound of meat and drink almost two gallons of raw milk each day during most of the year. Milk from the African Zebu cattle is much fattier than cow's milk, which means that the Samburus consume more than twice the amount of animal fat than the average American, and yet their cholesterol is much lower, about 170 mg/dl.

Heart disease should be blamed not on animal fats or cholesterol, but upon excess consumption of vegetable oils, hydrogenated fats, and refined carbohydrates; vitamin and mineral deficiencies; and the reduction or disappearance of antimicrobial fats from the food supply (from animal fats and tropical oils).

Most Crucial Fats for Health

The Maker's fats are essential for good health and maximum protection from disease. You find them in natural vegetable and animal sources. Many people do not realize that animal proteins and fats appear together for a reason—we need fat to properly assimilate protein and minerals. Perhaps our most important fats (and those we lack the most) are the omega-3 fatty acids found in cod liver oil, high-omega-3 eggs, and ocean-caught fish such as salmon, mackerel, and sardines. Small amounts are available in meat, poultry, and dairy products from grass-fed animals.

A word of caution: With the rising popularity of salmon, more and more distributors, grocery chains, and restaurants have turned to farm-raised salmon to meet demand, which is contrary to the Maker's design for salmon. Research has shown that the omega-3 fatty acids abundant in ocean-caught salmon are changed into omega-6 fatty acids when they are farm-raised, which creates an imbalance of these nutrients for your body. Always shop for ocean-caught salmon—especially the varieties from cold Alaskan waters, which offer a healthful balance of omega-3 and omega-6 fatty acids.

The liberal consumption of omega-3 fatty acids is crucial for negating the effects of the overabundance of omega-6 linoleic acids and hydrogenated fats present in most American diets—a combination linked to excess inflammation and tumor formation when in the presence of carcinogens and certain enzymes in cells lining the colon.

Beware of Hydrogenated Fats

Many hydrogenated fats (liquid fats injected with hydrogen gas at high temperatures under high pressure to make them solid at room temperature) are heavily promoted as "health foods," but scientific findings say otherwise. The production process converts them into indigestible trans-fatty acids, which is not good. Hydrogenated fats have been associated with cancer, atherosclerosis, diabetes, obesity, immune system dysfunction, low-birth-weight babies, birth defects, decreased visual acuity, sterility, difficulty in lactation, and problems with bones and tendons.

The Maker's Diet focuses on the balanced intake of natural fats occurring in ocean-caught fish, cod liver oil, omega-3 eggs, and grass-fed, organic, and free-range meats. It also includes animal products such as butter, cheeses, and full-fat lacto-fermented dairy products such as yogurt and kefir, as well as raw milk and cream from goats, sheep, cows, and other biblically clean mammals.

The Maker's Carbohydrates

Carbohydrates are the starches and sugars produced by all plants, synthesized by the body from proteins and fats, and refined by humans until they become "negative" calories that leach nutrients from the body rather than replace them.

Table sugar (sucrose) and its first cousin, refined and bleached wheat flour, are the stripped-down and nutrition-less versions of naturally occurring foods from nature. These refined products were virtually unknown before 1600 A.D., but they have certainly made their mark on the human race over the last four hundred years.

A Sugar Revolution

Sugar in all of its commercial forms has taken America by storm. Nearly two hundred years ago, the average American consumed about 10 pounds of sugar per year. Today, we gladly push aside healthier fare to gather fully one-fourth of our annual calorie intake from sugar—which is about 170 pounds of sugar each year for each and every one of us.

How would you like to see a grocery stock worker drop a heavy pallet of 170 one-pound bags of sugar beside your bed? Would you be willing to sit down and eat a bowl full of sugar every fourth meal—and nothing else? As bizarre as that may sound, according to the statistics, most of us are doing just that!

When two United Nations agencies—the World Health Organization (WHO) and the Food and Agriculture Organization—released the results of a study on how to halt the epidemic of obesity-linked diseases worldwide, they also issued a bold warning to reduce the percentage of sugar-based calories to no more than 10 percent.

Immediate protests and indignant news releases arose from the Sugar Institute (their news release carried the headline "Sugar Association Continues Disapproval of Release of Misguided WHO Diet and Nutrition Report"), the

Grocery Manufacturers of America (GMA), and the U.S. National Soft Drink Association, among others. I wonder why?

The saddest part of the picture for me is the official stance of the U.S. government—the leadership of a nation that leads the world in obesity. The U.S. government's "Dietary Guidelines for Americans" and official USDA guidelines include only a weak warning to consume sugar "in moderation"...while recommending fluoridated water as the preferred method of protecting teeth from cavities. And it directs the nation to consume even more carbohydrates from its USDA Food Guide Pyramid.

This is the same dietary picture and lifestyle that may put one out of every three Americans at risk of developing diabetes, according to K. M. Venkat Narayan, M.D., chief of the diabetes epidemiology section at the Centers for Disease Control in Atlanta. Meanwhile, the U.S. National Academy of Sciences' Institute of Medicine states that sugar could make up 25 percent of calories.

GRANDMA ROSE'S DIET

My Grandma Rose was born in 1922 on a Polish farm where they consumed fruits and vegetables straight from the garden; eggs from free-range chickens; dairy straight from the cow and goat; cold-water fish such as sardines; cod liver oil; and meats from grazing animals. They pressed flaxseed and poppy seed into oil, using their own mill.

"I used to eat lignan cakes as snacks with black sourdough bread," she told me one time. "We used to break off pieces from the flax cakes and dip them in fresh oil right from the press."

I'm convinced that Grandma's health problems began after her family emigrated to America in 1935, when she fell in love with white bread and ate a lot of junk food loaded with sugar, including cakes and doughnuts from the bakery. I can imagine that there are many similar stories of immigrants losing their health after coming to "the land of plenty."

A More Natural Way

The Maker's carbohydrates—including natural sugars—come directly from nature without so-called refinement or enrichment. There are two types of natural sugars found in carbohydrate foods. The first type consists of disaccharides, which are chains of two simple sugars. Disaccharides include sucrose (table sugar), lactose (milk sugar), maltose, and many others. Foods containing disaccharides include sugar, grains, potatoes, corn, and non-cultured dairy products. These foods can be difficult to digest unless they are consumed in their "predigested form," meaning they've been soaked, sprouted, and/or fermented.

The second type of sugar in carbohydrate foods consists of monosaccharides, which are simple or "single" sugars found in fruits, vegetables, nuts, seeds, fermented or sprouted grains, and dairy products. These are more easily digested. To eat carbohydrates the Maker's way, include only whole-grain products in your diet that have been properly treated through soaking, sprouting, or fermenting. These processes convert disaccharides to monosaccharides, which reduces or eliminates the phytates, or antioxidant compounds, that are not easily digested and can cause nutrient deficiencies.

These natural carbohydrates include wholesome whole-grain sourdough and sprouted-grain breads and cereal grains, soaked and fermented lentils, beans, and other legumes. They also include soaked seeds and nuts, fresh fruits and vegetables, and fermented vegetables.

Before the advent of mass-manufacturing processes, it was common for long-lived peoples to soak their grains overnight and allow them to dry in the open air until they were partially germinated or sprouted. Only then could they go through a leavening process. From these grains, ancient peoples made breads and pasta.

We now know these processes effectively remove the phytates from the outer covering of the natural grains. Phytates are substances that contain phosphorus in acidic form as well as powerful enzyme inhibitors that combine with (or "grab") minerals in the intestinal tract and block their absorption. Isn't it amazing that our ancestors prepared their food in a way that enhanced digestion and health, even though they had no scientific understanding at the time?

Some of the most toxic phytates appear in the extruded form of sugary breakfast cereals lining the shelves of America's grocery stores. According to Fallon and Enig, "Studies show that these extruded whole grain preparations can have even more adverse effects on the blood sugar than refined sugar and white flour!"

The late Dr. Edward Howell, one of the great enzyme scientists of the twentieth century and author of Food Enzymes for Health and Longevity, observed that the products of our "modern" mechanized harvesting techniques lack something our forefathers possessed in abundance—digestible or bioavailable nutrition.

Modern Techniques Decrease Nutrition Value

While modern techniques for harvesting crops definitely multiplied efficiency and greatly improved yields, these same techniques also decreased the nutrition value to the same degree. Dr. Howell, in his writings, described how the old harvesting techniques helped preserve and enhance the nutrition value of the grain. After cutting the mature grains in the field, farmers would gather the stalks and loosely bind them upright in sheaves and let them stand overnight in the field before threshing them—a process that removes the grain from the grass stalks—the following day. Threshing allowed the grains to germinate or sprout.

Germination, on the other hand, initiates a chemical transformation in the seed grains that naturally neutralizes the phytates or enzyme inhibitors the Creator put on the exterior of the seeds. When the seeds are activated or come alive, all of the nutrition within the seed becomes available for digestion. The germinated seeds of wheat and barley and the bread made from them were of great importance in biblical times. Called the "staff of life," bread supplied easily digestible, life-giving carbohydrates.

The big difference between then and now is that the people of the Bible didn't wolf down great quantities of carbohydrates like we do today. First of all, they ate significantly less food than we do today; the time between harvests could get awfully long. In fact, it was common for people in biblical times to eat only one meal a day at times. By today's standards, they consumed a lower-carbohydrate diet, and the grains they did eat were healthy, sprouted, or germinated with lower amounts of disaccharides and phytates.

The Maker's Dairy

One thing that hasn't changed since *The Maker's Diet* was released is the controversy over dairy products.

Eggs are bad for you; they have too much cholesterol.

Cow's milk is not suitable for human consumption.

Humans are the only mammals that consume milk after infancy.

Eggs are wonderful, nutrient-dense foods that pack six grams of protein, a bit of vitamin B-12, vitamin E, riboflavin, folic acid, calcium, zinc, and iron into a mere seventy-five calories. As for whether we should drink milk after infancy, the Bible makes it clear that milk produced by clean animals such as cattle, sheep, and goats is a viable food acceptable for human consumption.

The biggest problems with modern dairy products come from tinkering with dairy animals and their milk products to "make them better." Dairy farmers today selectively breed dairy cows and inject them with growth hormones to boost their annual milk production from 500 pounds to 3,000 pounds annually. That gives us lots of hormone-laced, antibiotic-rich milk for our enjoyment.

Rather than allow the cows to feed on grass in the field, it's cheaper and faster to pump them full of high-protein soybean meal. The cows, in turn, produce incredible amounts of milk for two years—and then suffer chronic mastitis (infections of the nipples) and shorter life spans. The milk we receive in such high quantities is very low in nutrients, especially when compared to the highly nutritious milk produced by grass-fed cows and other animals.

Fermentation and Unhealthy Milk Processing

Early and primitive societies understood the incredible value of milk products. Butter and cream, in particular, provided a treasure trove of vitamins, enzymes, and fats that promoted healthy bodies and long life. In the days before refrigeration, virtually every society practiced time-honored methods of fermentation to preserve and prepare dairy products for consumption over time.

You don't see fermentation going on today. Modern milk producers routinely pasteurize milk by heating it at high temperatures to destroy undesirable bacteria. This process destroys all of the beneficial organisms in milk, including 140 enzymes (which are considered the "final test" for successful pasteurization). Pasteurization also alters vital amino acids, reducing our ability to access the protein, fats, vitamins, and minerals in milk. In reality, modern sanitation standards, sterile, stainless steel holding tanks, and milking technology have made pasteurization largely unnecessary today.

Milk producers also add powdered milk and synthetic vitamin D2 or toxic D3 to low-fat milk to make it thicker. Then they homogenize the mixture so that fat particles remain in suspension, making them indigestible in the intestine but highly likely to pass through the intestinal wall and directly into the bloodstream.

Making Better Choices

Always choose butter over margarine or other low-fat spreads. Seek out raw goat's milk or raw cow's milk. It may be difficult, but an online search will be worth it.

Goat's milk in particular is very good for human consumption because it's easily digestible, digesting in only twenty minutes versus three hours for pasteurized cow's milk. Goat's milk contains less lactose (the type of sugar in milk that many find hard to digest) and is filled with vitamins, enzymes, and protein. If the idea of sipping from a glass of goat's milk has you turning up your nose, then let me remind you that 65 percent of the world's population drinks goat's milk.

Look for raw milk cheeses in health food stores, or learn how to make your own kefir, whole-milk yogurt, and other fermented dairy products if you're feeling industrious. The good news is that the fermentation process makes most dairy products very digestible for sensitive people.

The Maker's Fiber

For thousands of years, before the birth of corporate food giants, Americans ate foods barely one step from their natural state as the Creator intended. Vegetables were harvested from the garden just outside the back door, and fermented vegetables—packed in Mason jars—were enjoyed during the winter. Fruits were plucked from the family fruit trees and vines and also canned for consumption later.

The nutritious parts of these foods that could be digested were effectively passed through the intestinal wall into the bloodstream. The remainder—the fiber—consisting of the cell walls (cellulose), hemicellulose, pectin, lignans, gums, and mucilage that were indigestible continued the journey through the colon to final elimination.

Fiber: Friend or Foe

Fiber comes in two forms: insoluble and soluble.

Insoluble fiber cannot be broken down at all, while soluble fiber dissolves in water. Fiber is vital to the body because it promotes regular bowel movements, prevents constipation, increases the elimination of waste matter in the large intestine, and pressures the rectum muscles to loosen and expel waste without undue pressure on delicate rectal tissues.

Bran fiber became popular after a British missionary surgeon named Dr. Dennis Burkitt announced the results of pioneering studies in the 1970s in which he determined that rural Africans on high-fiber diets had far less colon cancer than people from the West. Dr. Burkitt had already distinguished himself by being the first to discover and describe what is now called "Burkitt's lymphoma" in 1958. His later discovery of a primitive people who had almost no diabetes, constipation, or irritable bowel syndrome seemed to support the conclusion that the Africans' high fiber intake accounted for their good intestinal health.

Dr. Burkitt's basic premise was right, in my opinion, but the American media and health culture took "the fiber hypothesis" in a totally different direction. While the African tribesmen Dr. Burkitt studied rarely ate grains, the idea was promoted in America that eating large amounts of bran fiber from whole-grain wheat would help prevent colon cancer, diverticulosis, hemorrhoids, and colonic polyps. Kellogg's successfully promoted their All-Bran cereal for these reasons.

For thirty years, the grain-fiber hypothesis (especially from bran) was considered the gospel truth. The truth, however, is that bran fiber actually aggravates many of these conditions. I couldn't eat bran fiber during my battle with Crohn's disease, and I won't touch it today due to the high amount of mineral-blocking phytates it contains.

Fiber found in grain is a carbohydrate. The overconsumption of high-carbohydrate grain-based foods such as bran, fibrous breakfast cereals, whole-wheat bread (nonsprouted or fermented), and soy, which all contain high amounts of phytates, is a primary cause of intestinal disease and other diseases.

Friendly Fiber

The Maker's recommended fiber sources—the kind of fiber that promotes colon health—are found in low-carbohydrate, high-fiber foods. These foods include broccoli, cauliflower, celery, and lettuce, as well as soaked or sprouted seeds, nuts, grains, and legumes. Berries and other small fruits, along with fruits and vegetables with edible skins, are also good sources of low-carbohydrate fiber. Besides providing the right kind of fiber, these foods are rich in vitamins, minerals, and antioxidants.

Another form of helpful fiber, called mucilaginous fiber, also helps relieve constipation and soothes inflamed tissue in the lining of the gut while decreasing transit time for proper elimination. Lowered transit times mean that toxins are quickly flushed out before they putrefy in the colon. Mucilaginous fiber is found in chia and flaxseeds.

The Maker's Fermentation

I once heard a health expert I respect say that the creation of the refrigerator was one of the worst inventions for our health. He didn't mean that it was a bad idea to keep milk, fruits, and vegetables cool so they don't spoil as rapidly. What he was lamenting was our lack of knowledge regarding fermented foods.

Before refrigeration, fermentation was the way everyone preserved food in a healthy way. Today, a hundred years later, few Americans from urban and suburban areas know anything about preserving food in this way. Most of the people in the world, however—including people in Asia, Africa, South America, and various Third World and emerging nations—still depend on fermentation to preserve foods and to protect them from dangerous organisms in other foods and drinks.

Thousands of years ago, Abraham served his best meat, dairy, and fermented cream curds to entertain his angelic visitors:

> So Abraham hurried into the tent to Sarah. "Quick," he said, "get three seahs of fine flour and knead it and bake some bread." Then he ran to the herd and selected a choice, tender calf and gave it to a servant, who hurried to prepare it. He then brought some curds and milk and the calf that had been prepared, and set these before them.
>
> —Genesis 18:6–8 (NIV)

It's said that the Chinese fermented cabbage as far back as six thousand years ago. And according to Annelies Schoneck, author of *Making Sauerkraut and Pickled Vegetables at Home*, the Roman emperor Tiberius always took a barrel of sauerkraut (fermented cabbage) with him when he made the long voyages to the Middle East. Fermentation is especially effective in releasing important nutritional compounds through pre-digestion that would otherwise pass through the human digestive system, undigested and unused.

Modern vinegar-based fermentation techniques used for large-scale commercial production do not produce the same benefits as lactic acid fermentation, which is driven by beneficial microorganisms. This natural biological activity produces enzymes that break down foods into usable compounds and inhibits putrefying bacterial growth.

Every long-lived culture in the world has consumed fermented vegetables, dairy, and meat. Aboriginal peoples of Australia buried sweet potatoes in the soil for months before removing and consuming them. The proliferation of lactobacilli and other friendly microorganisms in fermented vegetables enhances their digestibility, increases vitamin levels, and produces helpful enzymes as well as natural antibiotic and anti-carcinogenic substances.

The same thing occurs in lacto-fermented sauerkraut that's described in ancient Roman manuscripts, and in pickled green tomatoes, peppers, and lettuce in Russia and Poland. Asian peoples are known for their legendary pickled preparations of cabbage, turnip, eggplant, cucumber, onion, squash, and carrot, including Korean kimchi (a lacto-fermented condiment of cabbage with other vegetables and seasonings), and Japanese pickled vegetables.

American lacto-fermented foods include the full range of pickled vegetables, relishes, eggs, and many native fruits—plus nearly all of the fermented products from Europe, Asia, and nations south of the border. The problem is that Americans don't eat these fermented foods very often. We do better consuming lacto-fermented dairy products such as yogurt, kefir, cheeses, cottage cheese, and cultured cream (also called crème fraîche), which are exceptionally healthy and nutritious. (If you are lactose-intolerant, you should know that the healthful "probiotic" bacteria involved in the lacto-fermentation process feed on the lactose in milk, leaving behind galactose, an easily digested monosaccharide sugar.)

The Maker's Enzymes, Living Vitamins, and Minerals

When the Creator provided protein, He placed it in close proximity to healthy fats needed for proper assimilation of the protein. He also provided enzymes as a type of divine "match" to light the fires of digestion.

Enzymes are specialized proteins that trigger, facilitate, and accelerate chemical reactions, while remaining unchanged in the process. These natural catalysts are found in all living organisms, especially raw or uncooked food.

There are three types of enzymes: digestive, metabolic, and food enzymes. The three digestive enzymes are proteases (to digest protein), amylases (to digest carbohydrates), and lipases (to digest fat). These enzymes help the body break down food so it can be absorbed in the small intestine. The body itself manufactures metabolic enzymes that direct body functions and digestive enzymes.

Food enzymes are found only in uncooked raw foods. One such enzyme, cellulase, breaks down plant fiber known as cellulose and makes it digestible.

Cultural Enzyme Deficiency

Prolonged heat kills all enzymes, as does cooking, processing, and pasteurization. That is why we should eat raw foods along with our cooked foods. Lacto-fermented foods are especially rich in beneficial digestive enzymes of all types.

Dr. Howell, whom I mentioned earlier, maintained that every human being is born with a finite or fixed number of enzymes. Because these vital enzymes are limited, it is important to provide as many outside enzymes as possible from raw food sources. This is the central theme of his classic work Enzyme Nutrition.

Unfortunately, the vitamin and mineral content of American vegetables and fruits has declined over the last half century due to the overuse of fertilizers and other chemical additives, as well as mono-crop techniques that do not promote the natural replenishment of the soil. In addition, Americans are consuming fewer servings of even these less-potent fruits and vegetables, while loading up on junk food virtually devoid of all nutrients. This national eating pattern has produced widespread nutrient and enzyme deficiencies, thus leading to a number of health problems.

For many concerned individuals, the solution to nutritional deficiencies has been to turn to vitamin and mineral supplements. Unfortunately, what passes for vitamin and mineral supplements in grocery stores, pharmacies, and even health food stores often amounts to little more than lifeless isolated or synthetic chemicals. Worse yet, these laboratory-produced synthetic substitutes for food nutrients were never meant to be assimilated apart from their natural form in food.

Over 50 percent of the population take vitamin or mineral supplements to improve energy and performance and to reduce the risk of deadly diseases such as cancer, heart disease, and diabetes. Despite widespread use of vitamin and mineral supplements since their introduction only some seventy-five years ago, the incidence of those just-mentioned major diseases has skyrocketed. Even more surprising is the lack of scientific research showing the efficacy of multivitamin/mineral supplements.

I've always been a big fan of vitamins and minerals from soil-based organisms that resemble "living foods" and are in the natural form our Creator intended. These living foods supplements provide all of the necessary cofactors required for assimilation by the body, and they are literally "alive" with probiotics and enzymes.

Research conducted by Dr. Price led him to believe that without fat-soluble vitamin A (retinol) from animal sources such as butterfat, egg yolks, liver, and other organ meats, the body cannot utilize protein, minerals, or water-soluble vitamins. He also discovered what he called Activator X—or the X Factor—a fat-soluble nutrient that acts as a catalyst to mineral absorption. Activator X is found in cream from grass-fed animals, organic liver, and fish eggs.

In addition, there are seven "macro-minerals" (calcium, chloride, magnesium, phosphorus, potassium, sodium, and sulfur) and at least thirty trace minerals that are essential to life. If present in only minute amounts, these minerals prevent certain diseases and promote proper body function. The natural sources for minerals include nutrient-rich foods, beverages, broths, and living multivitamins with homeostatic nutrients.

The Maker's Top Healing Foods

More and more, history and science are confirming that the Creator's provisions for mankind's need for food are still the best choices for ensuring health and quality of life today. The following section reviews some of these top biblical foods that you can choose to include in your diet for health and longevity.

Fish and Fish Oil

If you follow the precise biblical recommendations for the Maker's seafood, you can ensure health and avoid disease. (See Leviticus 11:9–12.) Fish is a

wonderfully rich source of protein, potassium, vitamins, and minerals. For
those who simply don't get enough cold-water fish, it's imperative that you take
a form of high-quality cod liver oil every day. Today we understand scientifically that fish oil and cod liver oil:

* thin the blood
* protect the arteries from damage
* inhibit blood clots
* reduce blood triglycerides
* lower LDL blood cholesterol
* lower blood pressure
* reduce risk of heart attack and stroke
* ease symptoms of rheumatoid arthritis
* reduce risk of lupus
* relieve migraine headaches
* fight inflammation
* help regulate the immune system
* inhibit cancer in animals (and possibly humans)
* soothe bronchial asthma
* combat kidney disease

Much of the healing powers of fish reside in the omega-3 fatty acids that are
particularly concentrated in cold-water fish such as salmon, sardines, bluefish,
herring, mackerel, sablefish, whitefish, bluefin tuna, and anchovies, as well as
in the livers of cod.

Doctors in northern European countries like Iceland and Ireland have prescribed cod liver oil for more than two hundred years for a number of ailments,
including rheumatism and arthritis. Back then, it was believed that cod liver
could "lubricate the joints." It took until 1985 for doctors to officially recommend (in the New England Journal of Medicine) that arthritis sufferers could
benefit from eating fish once or twice a week, so one could say that omega-3
oils do lubricate the joints!

Three villains inside our bodies cause heart attacks and stroke:

* plaque, which can clog arteries and dangerously restrict blood
  flow

* the accumulation of platelets (sticky pieces of blood cells), which clump together and form clots
* the sudden, unexplained spasms of blood vessels, which can throw the heart out of kilter or halt the flow of blood to the brain, causing strokes

Studies show that cod liver oil high in omega-3 fats EPA and DHA reduces or eliminates all three risks. The higher the levels of omega-3 fatty acids in the blood, the lower your blood pressure and your risk of heart disease and cancer.

In study after study, cod liver oil has been acknowledged to play a role in the development of the brain, the rods and cones of the retina of the eye, the male reproductive tissue, skin integrity, lubrication of the joints, and the body's inflammatory response. This has made cod liver oil a recommended first-response treatment for early symptoms of autism and other neurological child-development problems.

Grains of the Bible: Barley and Wheat

God described the Promised Land as "a land of wheat and barley" (Deuteronomy 8:8). Was it coincidence that the young boy in John 6:9–13 brought Jesus five barley loaves with which He fed thousands? Barley has been consumed for thousands of years and is known to improve potency, vigor, and strength. Roman gladiators at times were called "barley eaters" because they ate barley before their contests for bursts of strength.

While barley and wheat can be valuable, their young sprouts—known as cereal grasses—are considered to be true miracle foods by many. These grasses contain four essential compounds largely absent from our diets:

1. antioxidant enzymes
2. trace minerals
3. chlorophyll
4. high-quality vegetable proteins

You can obtain the juice from young wheat and barley grasses by juicing them yourself or by consuming a green superfood powder containing the dried cereal grass juices.

Cultured Dairy from Goats, Cows, and Sheep

"You shall have enough goats' milk for your food, for the food of your household, and the nourishment of your maidservants," says Proverbs 27:27.

The milk consumed in biblical times differs a great deal from the milk we consume today. The milk of the Bible that came from cows and goats was consumed straight from the animal, meaning it was not pasteurized or homogenized, or it was immediately fermented. These "live" foods provide excellent health benefits in contrast to today's pasteurized, homogenized, often skimmed and fortified milk, which is not only less nutritious but also can be potentially harmful and a major cause of allergies.

It was virtually impossible to keep milk fresh in those days, so the people borrowed principles from the fermentation process used to make wine or sourdough bread to preserve their dairy products. The result was what we know today as yogurt, cheese (soft and hard), and what is sometimes called curds in the Bible (or butter curds in some translations). Here are some of the recently discovered health benefits of high-quality fermented dairy:

- fermented dairy provides calcium that builds bone in children and helps prevent or slow the development of osteoporosis that plagues so many elderly
- fermented dairy lowers high blood pressure and cholesterol
- fermented dairy attacks bacterial infections, especially those that cause diarrhea
- fermented dairy soothes stomach linings irritated from drugs or harsh foods
- fermented dairy prevents dental cavities and chronic bronchitis
- fermented dairy stops the growth of some cancers, including colon cancer
- fermented dairy boosts mental alertness and energy

High-quality fermented dairy can come from cow's or goat's milk. Many people find that they attain better results by consuming goat's milk rather than cow's milk because they can tolerate that form of dairy better. My research shows that goat's milk will digest in a baby's stomach in twenty minutes, whereas pasteurized cow's milk takes eight hours. The difference is in the structure of the milk.

Below are some of the health benefits attributed to goat's milk consumption:

* goat's milk is less allergenic because it does not contain the complex proteins that stimulate allergic reactions to cow's milk
* goat's milk does not suppress the immune system
* goat's milk is easier to digest than cow's milk
* goat's milk has more buffering capacity than over-the-counter antacids and more acid-buffering capacity than cow's milk, soy infant formula, and nonprescription antacid drugs
* goat's milk alkalinizes the digestive system
* goat's milk helps to increase the pH of the blood stream because it's the dairy product highest in the amino acid L-glutamine, an alkalinizing amino acid often recommended by nutritionists
* goat's milk contains twice the healthful medium-chain fatty acids such as capric and caprylic acids, which are highly antimicrobial
* goat's milk does not produce mucus and does not stimulate a defense response from the human immune system
* goat's milk is a rich source of the trace mineral selenium, a necessary nutrient known for its immune modulation and antioxidant properties

When consuming milk or yogurt, I usually recommend goat's milk sources, but high-quality dairy products from grass-fed cows can be excellent as well.

Olive Oil

The olive branch has symbolized peace throughout history, and olives and olive oil have been used as powerful remedies for a wide variety of ills.

Olive oil is one of the most digestible of all fats. A diet rich in olive oil contributes to longevity and reduces the wear and tear of aging on the body tissues, organs, and the brain. Consuming olive oil in your diet reduces the risk of heart disease and cancer and can protect you against stomach ulcers.

For all its health attributes, I believe high-quality extra-virgin olive oil should not be used in cooking, however, as some of the nutrients in olive oil become less effective when heated. I recommend that that olive oil be mixed into food once the food has cooled.

Small Fruit

Figs are mentioned more than fifty times in the Bible and are the first fruit specifically named in Scripture in Genesis 3:7. Whether fresh or dried, figs have been prized since ancient times for their sweetness and nutritional value.

Grapes were the first crop Noah planted after the flood (Genesis 9:20). They were made into wine and vinegar or eaten fresh or dried. We now know that grapes fight tooth decay, stop viruses in their tracks, and are rich in other ingredients that many researchers believe may lower risk of cancer.

Berries such as blueberries, strawberries, blackberries, and raspberries, while not mentioned explicitly in the Bible, are superfoods containing some of the highest levels of antioxidants known to man. Blueberries contain antioxidant compounds that show promise in reversing some of the effects of aging, especially cognitive function. Raspberries contain notable anti-carcinogenic compounds, are low in calories, and are high in fiber. They make a great addition to the diet.

Stocks and Soups

Stocks and soups appear in biblical diets, as we see in Judges 6:19, and meat and fish stocks are virtually universal fixtures in traditional cuisine in France, Italy, China, Japan, Africa, South America, Russia, and the Middle East. Chicken soup, widely considered a sure-fire cure for the common cold, is sometimes called "the Jewish penicillin." Fish soup enjoys the same reputation in the Orient and South America.

Properly prepared meat stocks are extremely nutritious and contain minerals, cartilage, collagen, and electrolytes all in an easily absorbable form. In addition, meat, fish, and chicken stocks contain generous amounts of natural gelatin, which aids digestion and helps heal many intestinal disorders, including heartburn, IBS, Crohn's disease, and anemia. Science has confirmed that broth helps prevent and mitigate infectious diseases.

Healthy Saturated Fats

Butter from grass-fed cows, extra-virgin coconut oil, and animal fats have nourished human beings for several thousand years. For the last five decades, though, Americans avoided these fats based on erroneous advice and increased their consumption of polyunsaturated and hydrogenated fats instead.

As I've mentioned earlier, the rate of heart disease has increased, as has obesity and many immune system disorders despite this advice. I believe it's time to return to healthy fats from whole, grass-fed cow butter from properly raised animals and extra-virgin coconut oil.

Whole-milk butter produced from cows eating rapidly growing green grasses is loaded with vitamins A, D, and E. It's also high in Activator X, which significantly increases the effectiveness of vitamin A's ability to stimulate a person's immune system, as described by Dr. Weston Price. Whole-milk butter also contains a healthy balance of omega-6 to omega-3 fatty acids, as well as conjugated linoleic acid, or CLA. (These characteristics are seriously compromised once a cow has any grain introduced to its diet.)

CLA is strictly a product of bacterial function and is virtually nonexistent in cow-milk fat during any period when grain is in the diet. For many types of cancer, CLA 9-11 has been proven to prevent and retard tumor cell growth.

The quality of Activator X and other vitamins is directly related to the quality of the grass and forage the cow is eating. The faster the grass is growing when the cow is grazing it, the higher the vitamin content. Make sure to buy butter from grass-fed cows. The first telltale sign that the butter you are consuming is from grass-fed cows is its yellow color.

Extra-virgin coconut oil is one of the healthiest saturated fats available. Don't listen to the misguided advice of so-called health experts warning against the saturated tropical oils such as coconut and palm oils. Coconut oil can tolerate extremely high heat, unlike polyunsaturated vegetable oils. Use extra-virgin coconut oil in cooking, baking, and in smoothies. This stable, healthy saturated fat does not elevate undesirable (LDL) cholesterol and reduces the symptoms of digestive disorders, supports overall immune functions, and helps prevent bacterial, viral, and fungal infections.

Extra-virgin coconut oil is great for women suffering from Candida yeast infections, due to the presence of caprylic acid and anti-fungal fatty acids contained in the oil. Extra-virgin coconut oil has also been shown to help balance the thyroid and improve metabolic function, which may result in weight loss.

Honey

The Creator also chose to use honey to describe the abundance of the Promised Land, telling the Israelites that they were about to enter the land of "milk and honey" (Exodus 13:5). Honey is one of the most powerful healing foods we have at our disposal. Generations of grandmothers have prepared hot honey drinks to soothe sore throats, calm frayed nerves, and ensure a good night's sleep. Asthmatics often swear by honey's ability to help them breathe easier. Honey wipes out bacteria that cause diarrhea and may eliminate such disease-causing bacteria as salmonella, Shigella, E. coli, and cholera.

The Bible implies a strong influence of butter and honey on brain function. "Curds [butter] and honey He shall eat, that He may know to refuse the evil and choose the good," says Isaiah 7:15 (KJV). The brain is made of mostly fat (which butter provides), and it runs on glucose (of which honey is an excellent source). Always look for high-quality honey produced locally and sold in its raw and unheated form—this preserves its rich storehouse of naturally occurring enzymes and bee pollen.

Pomegranate

Pomegranate is called the fruit of royalty in the Bible and is one of the richest sources of antioxidants. Pomegranates contain high amounts of ellagic acid, an antioxidant with proven anticancer properties and excellent benefits for female health.

Wild Animal Foods

Grass-fed red meat, poultry, and wild game have nourished humans for thousands of years. Grass-fed beef, buffalo, lamb, goat, and venison are valuable sources of nutrients that protect and enhance the immune and circulatory systems. They contain cysteine, glutathione, coenzyme Q10, carnitine, MSM, CLA, several B vitamins, zinc, magnesium, and vitamins A and D as well as omega-3 fatty acids.

Properly raised red meats provide an excellent source of complete proteins. Lamb and goat represent two of nature's best sources of carnitine, a fat-soluble nutritional factor that helps drive fatty acids into the cells for energy use. (Carnitine supplements are standard therapy for congestive heart failure and high triglycerides, and they are helpful during recovery after a heart attack.) Free-range pastured chicken, turkey, and duck are good sources of protein, fatty acids, and fat-soluble vitamins. Chicken and turkey contain generous amounts of tryptophan, a natural sedative.

Seeds (Soaked and Sprouted)

These rich sources of nutrients become real nutritional powerhouses when they are soaked and sprouted. The germination process (sprouting) produces vitamin C and increases carotenoids and vitamin B content, especially B2, B5, and B6. Even more importantly, sprouting neutralizes phytic acid, a substance present in the bran of all seeds that inhibits the absorption of calcium, magnesium, iron, and zinc.

Sprouting also neutralizes enzyme inhibitors present in all seeds. This is important, because these inhibitors can neutralize our own precious enzymes in the digestive tract, which is one reason many people seem to get a stomachache or excess gas after consuming large amounts of seeds. Sprouting can also inactivate certain toxins found in seeds.

Omega-3 Eggs

High omega-3 eggs are nature's nearly perfect food. Eggs contain all known nutrients except for vitamin C! They are good sources of fat-soluble vitamins A and D as well as certain carotenoids that guard against free-radical damage to the body. They also contain lutein, which has been shown to prevent age-related macular degeneration. When possible, buy eggs directly from farms where the chickens are allowed to roam free and eat their natural diet, or purchase eggs marked DHA or high omega-3 eggs.

Despite the unfounded cholesterol scare of the last twenty years, eggs can be a healthy addition to anyone's diet.

Cultured/Fermented Vegetables

Fermented vegetables such as sauerkraut, pickled carrots, beets, or cucumbers are some of the most health-giving foods on the planet. Raw cultured or fermented vegetables provide the body with beneficial microorganisms known as probiotics and an abundance of enzymes.

They are also a rich source of many vitamins, including vitamin C, and are very easy to digest. Sauerkraut (fermented cabbage) contains nearly four times the cancer-fighting nutrients as unfermented cabbage and is the primary source of vegetable nutrition in many countries where the winters are cold.

Cultured/fermented vegetables are very easy to make and are readily available at health food stores everywhere.

Organ Meats

Although native peoples have always prized the inner organs of game and domestic animals, irrational and unscientific fears about cholesterol have driven organ meats, like liver and heart, out of Western diets. Organ meats are the most nutrient-dense part of animals, but even natural health authorities routinely tell people not to eat organ meats for fear of consuming toxins found in these organs (especially liver).

It is true that the liver filters toxins from the body, but the benefits derived from consuming liver from organically raised, grass-fed animals far outweigh any negatives. Liver is one of nature's richest sources of vitamins A, D, B6, B12, folic acid, iron, glutathione, and various fatty acids. Raw liver figures prominently in many world-renowned alternative cancer protocols, including the Kelley and Gerson programs.

Fermented Beverages

It is difficult to think of popular modern beverages that qualify as healthy beverages. It is time to return to the lacto-fermented beverages that have supplied beneficial probiotics, enzymes and minerals, rapid hydration, and enhanced digestion to people throughout the world. Some typical fermented beverages include kefir, grape cooler, natural ginger ale as well as kombucha and kvass.

These lactic-acid-containing drinks help relieve intestinal problems, including constipation, and promote lactation, strengthen the sick, and promote overall well-being and stamina. They are considered superior to plain water in their ability to relieve thirst during physical labor. Many scholars believe that the "new wine" consumed in the Bible was a nonalcoholic lacto-fermented beverage.

Green Vegetables

Green leafy vegetables are some of the most nutrient-dense foods on the planet, including many nutrients not found in any other foods. Greens contain large amounts of beta carotene and virtually every mineral and trace element.

Many experts believe that ideally we should be consuming between three and five servings of green leafy vegetables per day.

If you can't get enough greens from food, try juicing fresh greens or supplementing with a powdered green superfood drink containing dried juices of wheat and barley grass and other vegetables. Your Creator knows better than anyone does what makes your body function at its peak capacity while remaining free of disease. He designed the bounty of the earth and a wide variety of foods to be the cornerstone of a long and healthy life.

The first and most dramatic step anyone can make toward renewed or greater health is to return to the Maker's Diet, which is based on the sound nutrition principles given to us in the Scriptures. Your Creator is also vitally concerned with the spirit and soul living inside your body. He knows that you are not just what you eat—you are also what you think.

9

You Are What You Think

From the moment the Creator planted the first human in the middle of an incredibly complex creation, we have scrambled to accumulate, organize, analyze, categorize, label, and understand knowledge about the universe surrounding us.

Because we are finite or limited creatures, we must break things down into bite-sized portions to learn and understand them. It's critical to consider how we perceive our universe and our personal world, for that perception—or worldview—will largely determine our existence.

During and after the Reformation, and especially during the twentieth century, it became popular among certain intellectuals to dismiss the spiritual side of the human race in favor of two broad philosophical viewpoints:

1. We are purely animal life forms operating solely as highly evolved organisms driven by chemical reactions.
2. We are life forms with highly advanced mental capacities that have "evolved" into more or less "spiritual" beings, creating our own gods as we need them.

Neither of these views of mankind is expressed in the Scriptures, and they have produced tremendous problems as these beliefs have infiltrated the scientific and philosophical communities, gradually influencing the way we perceive life and approach physical, mental, and even spiritual issues.

For example, some psychiatrists view humans as simply chemical or organic beings whose every mental state is created by or dramatically influenced by chemical reactions. Therefore, in their view, every mental malady we face can be isolated to chemical imbalances and "fixed with a pill." This godless way of thinking is demeaning and narrow-minded at best. The Scriptures warn:

> The fool says in his heart, "There is no God."...The Lord looks down from heaven on the sons of men to see if there are any who understand, any who seek God.
>
> —PSALM 14:1A–2 (NIV)

God created us in His image (Genesis 1:27), and God is a Spirit (John 4:24). Therefore, we are spirit beings who have souls (a mind, a will, and emotions) and who live in physical bodies. Our "parts" cannot be divided without skewing or misunderstanding the whole.

God made you a complex, interrelated being, fully integrated and interdependent. Even alternative and holistic health practitioners fall into the same error often made in conventional medicine—they try to fix one system or function instead of addressing the whole person: spirit, soul, and body.

I'm convinced that the Creator knew what He was doing when He created us, and I believe His Word is the foundation for total health: spiritual, mental, and emotional, as well as physical. I'm thankful for science and human advances in medicine and nutrition, but when science dismisses the Creator's foundational principles, I'm certain that His pattern provides us with a better approach to life.

We must emphasize the whole being—body, soul, and spirit—and provide the individual with all of the tools needed to maintain or recapture complete health and wholeness.

It is clear from Scripture that in each person, spirit, soul, and body are very closely linked. The computer science concept GIGO (garbage in, garbage out) may best describe the most crucial "equation" available for the human condition. You and I are not computers, but the formula really does apply to virtually every area of human existence. If you allow "garbage" into your body, mind, or spirit, you can expect to "express" garbage. In fact, I have it on the highest authority:

> For as he thinks in his heart, so is he. "Eat and drink!" he says to you, but his heart is not with you.
>
> —PROVERBS 23:7 (NKJV)

For whatever is in your heart determines what you say. A good person produces good words from a good heart, and an evil person produces evil words from an evil heart.

—MATTHEW 12:34–35 (NLT)

As examples of modern ways to entertain "garbage," consider the following scenarios:

* If you eat junk food, excessive amounts of sugar and preservatives, and favor the unclean foods the Creator warned us about, then you will almost certainly reap an unpleasant harvest of failed health later in life.
* If your friends and close associates are people who use recreational drugs, abuse prescription drugs, get drunk, and are promiscuous, then you're likely to fall into a dangerous lifestyle yourself sooner or later.
* If you fill your mind with unhealthy and unwholesome images of pornography, violence, fractured relationships, and scornful attitudes about God, eternal values, and godly living, you will begin to act out what you put in.

What You Do Starts with What You Think

In most cases, the things you do and say begin with the things you think and believe. You are barraged by stressing circumstances and challenges every day. How do you deal with them? Do you even try?

Imagine your life as a glass filled to the halfway mark with water. How would you describe the way your life is going? Is the glass half full, or is the glass half empty? Your answer may reveal a lot about your thought life and worldview. A positive view would say "half full," considering what you have; a negative view would say "half empty," focusing on what you don't have.

So where do you fall? Or are you too stressed out to think about it?

Stress is a natural part of life; some experts say that stress is life. Psychologist and author Dr. Kevin Leman said the best definition for stress he has ever found was this: Stress is the "wear and tear on our bodies produced by the very process of living." He explained that stress comes from good things as well as bad circumstances, but trouble comes when stressful living lingers for days and weeks. "It reminds me of buying the best DieHard battery you can find, but if you have a habit of leaving the lights on, even a DieHard finally runs down," Leman said.

Develop Your Stress Management Skills

Stress comes at you from at least four sources:

1. Outward circumstances over which you have *no* control
2. Circumstances or influences over which you *do* have control
3. Inward attitudes, beliefs, and thought patterns
4. Internal physical conditions

For maximum health, it's important to become skilled in handling stress according to the Creator's principles.

According to Dr. Michael D. Jacobson, author of The Word on Health, cortisol and DHEA are two of the most critical stress hormones produced by your body. Cortisol is a steroid hormone that affects your body in ways similar to prednisone, meaning it blocks inflammation and suppresses the immune system.

DHEA is the balancing hormone that reverses the effects of cortisol. (DHEA has anti-aging effects, boosts the immune system, and exerts key influence on sex hormones—and thus, fertility.) Both are produced by the adrenal cortex, which is directly affected by your brain.

One of the important keys to achieve a healthy life is to eat a diet and live a lifestyle that promotes a healthy balance of DHEA and cortisol. When the two hormones are in balance, we experience excellent health physically, mentally, and emotionally.

The adrenals also produce the neurotransmitters adrenaline and noradrenaline and help regulate blood pressure as well as salt and water balance through the production of aldosterone, an anti-diuretic hormone. Excess adrenaline can wreak havoc on the human digestive system, skin, heart and circulatory system, and mental state. Excess cortisol, with its powerful immunosuppressive powers, may even open the door to runaway infection, cancer, hyperthyroidism, poor wound healing, diabetes, infertility, and mental instability.

Anger, resentment, unforgiveness, and a desire for revenge all trigger the classic "alarm triad" response to stress, which involves adrenal gland hypertrophy (swelling) and thymus and lymph gland atrophy (shrinkage), which indicates the suppression of the immune system and gastric inflammation.

Is It Really Worth It?

These age-old "life-shorteners" were well documented in Scripture long before scientists and researchers set out to quantify the effects of negative emotions on our bodies. At last we are beginning to catch up to the Creator's wisdom. Is it really worth the dangerous cost to hold on to anger or unforgiveness? Are we really willing to destroy ourselves in a quest for revenge?

When it comes to stress, it seems that the body can handle the day-to-day emergencies and surprises without any problem—but when stress hangs on, it drains the adrenal system like a car battery when the lights have been left on all night, making a "crash" inevitable.

In contrast, studies have shown that people "who experienced an episode of deep appreciation or love for five minutes saw their IgA levels [an antibody secreted in saliva and other body fluids as a first line of defense against infection] rise to 40 percent above normal and stay elevated for six hours," said Dr. Jacobson in his book.

Even simple lifestyle adjustments can make a significant difference in your stress levels.

- If you feel too busy to get away from your smartphone, then your stress-buster may be setting your phone to vibrate—or turning it off completely.
- If you usually eat on the run, choose to sit down when you eat and turn off your smartphone or TV. Don't allow your thoughts to be occupied with worry, irritation, or uncertainty. Focus on your meal and on pleasant thoughts. I recommend conversation with good friends during meals or reading something uplifting, such as God's Word.
- Get proper rest. There's simply no substitute for quality sleep. Sleep is so vital to good health that I often refer to sleep as the most important non-nutrient you can get.

The Deadly Stress of Fear

Unmanaged stress can kill you and may be the single most important trigger of heart attacks. A 2014 study of over 17,000 found that long-term exposure to the threat of terrorism can elevate people's resting heart rates and increase their risk of dying. This statistics-based study, performed by the Hebrew University of Jerusalem, is the largest of its kind and indicated that fear, induced by consistent exposure to the threat of terror, can lead to negative health consequences and increase the risk of mortality.

Studies like this mirror traumatic, stressful events in the past that impacted the health of those living through them. A report in the Journal of Clinical Basic Cardiology said that sudden cardiac deaths increased significantly during the Northridge earthquake in California in 1994 and in the Israeli civilian population during the first days of the Gulf War in 1991 when Saddam Hussein of Iraq rained down Scud missiles onto the Tel Aviv populace. A 58 percent increase in mortality from cardiovascular diseases was noted on the day of the first strike on Israel by Scud missiles. Female death rates increased 77 percent, while male mortality increased 41 percent.

These days around the globe, the fear of terrorism is real, and the effects of fear on the body confirm the very real link between the spirit, soul (mind and emotions), and body. Closer to home, where we are presumably safer, some experts have estimated that stress accounts for as much as 75 percent of all visits to a physician!

Beware the Dangerous Unity of Dysfunction

I'm persuaded that we help create many of our problems through wrong thinking, poor decision making, and poor dietary choices. When these factors unite and start working against us, sickness or death usually isn't far behind. The problem of arteriosclerosis perfectly illustrates this kind of dangerous "unity" in dysfunction.

Arteriosclerosis is a generic term for several vascular diseases in which the arterial wall becomes thickened and loses elasticity. The most common and serious form of atherosclerosis involves fat deposits on blood vessel walls.

Vascular disease, which affects the brain, heart, kidneys, other vital organs, as well as the extremities, is the leading cause of death in the U.S. and the world. Just over 800,000 people in the U.S. die each year from cardiovascular diseases. Stroke kills nearly 129,000 people, and about 116,000 people die of a heart attack each year, according to the Centers for Disease Control and Prevention and other governmental sources. The number of deaths from cardiovascular disease alone is one of every three deaths in America and accounts for more lives than all forms of cancer combined.

Sudden stress is the most common trigger for fatal heart attacks because it's able to crack the smooth covering of plaque common in people with atherosclerosis. This sets off a fatal chain reaction in the blood vessel that becomes clogged with plaque, which then dams up or shuts off blood flow to the heart—triggering a heart attack.

Anyone—whether he or she is a health-conscious individual or a health professional—who doubts the effect of the thought life on physical well-being should consider the list of diseases caused or worsened by emotional stress. This list was compiled by S.I. McMillen, M.D., and David E. Stern, M.D., in their landmark book None of These Diseases, and is the result of twenty-eight separate medical research studies and texts specifically offered as references for doctors, students, and researchers seeking further proof.

In their thesis statement, Doctors McMillen and Stern declared that emotional stress causes or worsens the following health problems:

* digestive system disorders
* circulatory system disorders
* genito-urinary systems disorders
* nervous system disorders
* glandular disorders
* allergies and immune system problems
* inflammation of muscles and joints
* infections
* inflammatory and skin diseases
* cancer

If you or someone you love suffers from any of the conditions on that list, let me reassure you that there is hope. As depressing as the facts about stress may appear, you do not have to become a victim of tension and worry! Countless numbers of people have overcome the negative effects of stress in the worst possible situations. In fact, Dr. McMillen nearly died of a bleeding ulcer before he learned how to successfully manage the stress in his life. His near-death crisis inspired the writing of the classic book *None of These Diseases*, in which he wrote this:

> Our reaction to stress is an important key to longer, better living. When we feel stressed out, will we give up or keep going? Will we see it as an irritation or a challenge? Will we blow a fuse or let it charge us up? We hold the key. We can decide whether stress will work for us or against us—whether stress will make us better or bitter.

Negative Thoughts, Negative Words

In his book *What You Don't Know May Be Killing You*, Don Colbert, M.D., described the story of a Jewish Holocaust survivor during World War II from Warsaw, Poland. When the Nazis discovered that he spoke German, they forcibly separated him from his wife, two daughters, and three sons because they could use him to deal with the prisoners. Then the SS guards mowed his family down with machine guns right in front of his eyes.

Author and psychiatrist George Ritchey was with the American troops who liberated the death camp survivors—including this man. Ritchey described this man's life in Return from Tomorrow: "For six years he had lived on the same starvation diet, slept in the same airless and disease-ridden barracks as everyone else, but without the least physical or mental deterioration." This miraculous survivor had no control over his outward circumstances and shared the same misery inflicted on millions of Jewish victims, yet he still survived.

What was his secret? He told Dr. Ritchey, "I had to decide...whether to let myself hate the soldiers who had done this...I had seen, too often, what hate could do to people's minds and bodies. Hate had just killed the six people who mattered most to me in the world. I decided then that I would spend the rest of my life, whether it was a few days or many years, loving every person I came into contact with."

When his camp was liberated, this man immediately didn't think of his welfare first. He went to work with the liberators, working fifteen to sixteen hours per day serving his fellow death camp survivors. Dr. Colbert observed, "He had learned the secret that negative thoughts lead to negative words, which lead to negative attitudes and emotions."

A Vital Key: Remove Negativity

One of the keys to my recovery was removing negative thinking and negative statements from my life. When I flew to San Diego to live with Bud Keith, the man who taught me the first principles of how to eat foods from the Bible, he forced me to examine my negative thinking. Basically, Bud did that by giving me no choice.

I stayed in his home with his wife and children, and he would not tolerate any negativity. I used to sit on his living room couch wearing a frown, which had become a regular part of my wardrobe for two years. He eventually banished me to my bedroom because he didn't want his kids to learn my negative demeanor from me! His tough standards of conduct amounted to a rough boot camp for my soul.

I had no one to complain to because the family was not allowed to entertain negative words. It wasn't long before the positive principles he taught started wearing off on me.

One time, as I was leaving the bathroom, I remember thinking, I may have another stomachache in ten minutes, but right now I'm fine, so I'm healed. I started believing my positive statement and thanking God for my healing. From that point on, I learned to count my blessings for the few moments that I had when I was free from pain and nausea. Right from the get-go, I learned a valuable lesson in how to live a moment-to-moment life of thanksgiving.

One night, after several weeks on the biblical diet, I decided that I would no longer focus on the negative or on what would happen tomorrow or in the next hour. I took conscious steps to make the change from negativity to thinking positive thoughts, but it was worth it! If I could only say positive things (which were all that were allowed in that home), I had to find the positive in any seemingly negative situation, like those moments early on when I didn't feel agonizing pain. I'd say, "I'm well for this moment," and let it go at that. That's when I discovered that faith is not just something you say—it's something you live, moment by moment.

The impact of this change in my thinking was a huge factor in my healing. I believe that faith and positive thinking, based on God's Word, are vital keys to recovering and maintaining health. That is why faith the size of a tiny mustard seed can move mountains. (See Matthew 17:20.) Even when I was sick and unhappy, I tried to have faith that I would get better. That was the seed—or foundation—from which my miracle could "grow."

Psychologist Dan Baker discovered virtually the same thing after dealing with the devastating death of his infant son, Ryan. The author of *What Happy People Know* said after his son's death that he "wanted to wrestle with God and rewrite history."

"Happy people are hugely resilient on the whole," he wrote. "One thing happy people know is that they don't get to be happy all the time. They can appreciate the moments, the little victories, the small miracles, and the relationships with one another."

The Placebo Effect

It's a commonly known fact that approximately three out of every ten people will see their symptoms change significantly if they believe they have received a valuable treatment for a physical condition. In fact, researchers count on this happening every time they conduct a scientific, double-blind study.

Dr. Michael Jacobson explained the phenomenon this way:

> In a typical study, it is expected that around one-third of the placebo group [the group of subjects who receive a "sugar pill" or fake treatment exactly like the real dose] will actually show as much benefit as if they were on the actual medication. This improvement may be due simply to the positive physical changes that can take place when a person believes that he is getting better.

The placebo effect is especially strong with people who have no anchor of absolute truth and faithfulness in their lives. Personally, I'm convinced that if one hundred healthy people were told by a physician they had incurable cancer and had only six months to live, approximately thirty of them would die. That's how powerful faith or the power to believe, even in the negative, can be.

The placebo effect is yet another indication pointing to the power of our thoughts over our physical condition. I'm not advocating a kind of "mind-over-matter" therapy here, but this phenomenon gives us a hint about the marvelous tool for health and power that God has given us in the human mind. It's no wonder the apostle Paul said that we should take every thought captive. (See 2 Corinthians 10:5.)

At the time I wrote the original *Maker's Diet,* two Danish researchers questioned the validity of the placebo phenomenon. In a report entitled, "Are 'Dummy Pills' a Dumb Idea, or Do They Really Help?", their findings questioned the effect of placebos outside of their use as a baseline for comparison in clinical trials. In a pointed response, John Bailar III, M.D., Ph.D., found faults with the study and called the negative conclusions "too sweeping."

The fact is, most doctors know a treatment is sometimes useless but because many patients demand some sort of medication for their condition, they oblige. For example, they routinely prescribe antibiotics for a flu bug because of the patient's expectation that he or she will walk out of the examination with something to take to the local pharmacy. The downside to this practice is that the indiscriminate use of antibiotics kills all bacteria, both good and bad, which can leave the patient even more vulnerable to a bug making the rounds.

Placebo Versus Faith

Dr. Jacobson made a big distinction between the placebo effect and the power of faith—and so do I. The placebo effect is based on a person's belief in the treatment and cannot be attributed to the properties of the placebo itself, a firm conviction regarding the absolute truth of God and His eternal Word.

In my search for health, I had plenty of opportunities to experience the placebo effect. After all, each of the seventy doctors and health practitioners informed me that they sure their "cure" would work for me; otherwise, they would not have suggested this course of treatment. Based on the treatment plans they presented me, it's natural that I would put my trust in their ability to help me feel better.

None of them ever helped me. Instead, it took faith in God's Word—and obedience to it—to really trigger a turnaround in my life.

Faith is powerful, and it produces hope. Hope begins with knowing that your Creator cares about you and that He has a plan for your life. This was one of my favorite Scriptures when I was going through my health issues:

> *"For I know the plans I have for you," declares the Lord, "plans to prosper you and not to harm you, plans to give you hope and a future."*
> —JEREMIAH 29:11 (NIV)

Hope is a big deal. Doctors McMillen and Stern noted a Harvard Medical School Conference in which a study was reviewed documenting that weekly churchgoers in Maryland were less likely than people who didn't attend church regularly to die from heart attacks (50 percent), emphysema (56 percent), cirrhosis (74 percent), and suicide (53 percent). Similar results were found in studies of different population groups at three different medical teaching universities.

I submit that it was the hope we have in Christ to never forsake us that helped the Maryland churchgoers live healthier lives.

The Power of Prayer

All of the great heroes of the Bible, from Abraham to Hannah (the mother of the prophet Samuel), to John the Beloved (the author of the one of the four gospels as well as the Book of Revelation), all were people of fervent faith and devotion. One after another, they demonstrated the power and peace available through prayer and communion with the Creator of all.

People of faith have known the truth regarding the power in prayer since time began. Now, even the secular worlds of psychology and medicine are finally catching on. Studies are popping up all the time promoting the power of prayer (or meditation). Hospitals across the land have bolstered their "prayer therapy" for the sick and recovering.

Biblical prayer incorporates more than words—it often includes the healing touch of caring people of faith, and the results are often nothing less than miraculous. In the very least, they are comforting in times of need.

The Healing Power of Laughter

The Bible tells us, "A merry heart does good, like medicine, but a broken spirit dries the bones" (Proverbs 17:22, NKJV). Dr. Don Colbert noted that research conducted by the Department of Behavioral Medicine at the UCLA Medical School into the physical benefits of happiness proved conclusively that "laughter, happiness, and joy are perfect antidotes for stress."

Dr. Colbert added this: "A noted doctor once said that the diaphragm, thorax, abdomen, heart, lungs—and even the liver—are given a massage during a hearty laugh."

Dr. Michael Miller from the University of Maryland told attendees at an American Heart Association Conference, "We don't know why laughter protects the heart...We know that exercising, not smoking and eating foods low in saturated fat, will reduce the risk of heart disease. Perhaps regular hearty laughter should be added to the list."

Dr. Miller added this in an interview with the BBC: "The [doctor's] recommendations for a healthy heart may one day be exercise, eat right, and laugh a few times a day."

Here's my professional opinion about the whole thing: "You gotta laugh a little!"

Moral of the Story

Here's the moral of this chapter: When I started to believe I was getting well in San Diego and gave thanks to God for the moments of well-being I was experiencing, I began to feel better and get well. That memorable moment when I asked my mother to take my picture at 111 pounds, when I was barely able to stand, demonstrated the seed of faith that sparked my healing. It was that mustard seed of faith that eventually moved the mountain of illness in my life.

A seemingly far-fetched, ridiculous-sounding, positive thought, word, or action that you can choose to express in your moment of desperation can act as a seed of faith that will spark the healing process for you. As you meditate on God's Word and pray, daring to quote His promises for your healing, your faith will grow, and you will receive your miracle as I received mine.

≈

10

Stop, Drop, and Roll!

ELEMENTARY SCHOOLCHILDREN HEAR IT OVER AND OVER AGAIN: "IF your clothing catches fire, immediately stop, drop, and roll!" This fire safety formula has a genuine application to the problem of physical, mental, and spiritual burnout as well.

When it comes to your health, if you sense the heat of life on your backside and smell the smoke of imminent burnout billowing around you, just stop, drop, and roll—or, more literally, *rest, fast, and exercise.*

Just as an automotive manufacturer provides detailed information and maintenance schedules for sustaining maximum performance and utility of your car, so your Creator has provided detailed instructions and maintenance schedules for preserving peak performance for you. Even if your friends confuse you with the Energizer bunny, you still need regular periods of rest.

Stop: We All Need a Sabbath Rest

Every working creature needs a Sabbath rest—and that goes for people, animals, and even farmland! People and animals need a break every seven days, and soil prospers with a break at least every seven years. Every wise farmer understands the need to put fields and crops in rotation so that the soil can replenish at least one growing season every seven years. Unfortunately, the trend with Big Agriculture is to plant the same crop year after year in the same fields, a practice that has greatly depleted our topsoil as well as the nutrients in our vegetables and fruits.

Dr. Mark Virkler, author of *Eden's Health Plan—Go Natural,* cited a study comparing two identical farming soils. One was farmed continuously for eight years while the other was allowed to stand fallow or not farmed. The soil from the field that had no Sabbath rest contained 1,097 parts per million (ppm) nutritional solids, while the fallow or rested field soil yielded an astounding 2,871 ppm of nutritional solids. That is two-and-a-half times more nutritional solids than the over-farmed soil!

Another author, Elmer Josephson, noted that the anti-God rebels who seized the reins of France during the bloody French Revolution of 1789 decided to increase the entire nation from a seven-day workweek—with Sundays off—to a ten-day cycle before a day of rest. Before long, the nation's horses and mules became diseased and died at alarming rates. After scientists investigated, they found that a return to the seventh day principle was necessary to physical welfare, health, and long life. "As someone has said, 'The donkeys taught the atheists a lesson in practical theology,'" Josephson wrote in *God's Key to Health and Happiness*.

Rest is crucial to the health of your body and soul, and sleep is an absolute and undeniable necessity of life. Lengthy and regular periods of rest are equally important over the long haul. Europeans are far ahead of Americans in this area. By my observation, it is normal for many European families to take extended vacations each year for periods averaging between four and six weeks! Most Americans struggle just to take a two-week vacation every year, and many who aren't full-time employees (or have two or more part-time jobs) take no vacation because they don't accrue a vacation pay benefit.

Besides giving us the night for regular sleep, the Creator programmed people and animals to rest completely every seventh day. You rest by stopping all labor—including the mental labor that has been proven to be more exerting to the adrenal system and the entire body than physical labor. (And that mental labor includes looking at your smartphone every ten minutes.)

When we tinker with His design, things start to unravel. Remember, even the Creator rested on the seventh day.

Do You Need a Good Reboot?

One of the first things I learned about computers and smartphones was that many of the seemingly serious problems could be "fixed" by turning it off and turning it back on. This allows the software to "reboot" and start all over again. So it is with the body. When you reboot, you stop, rest, and start all over again.

Drop (Your Fork): Fasting

It's a great idea to give your body's digestive system a rest, too. This is what the Bible calls fasting.

Biblical leaders such as David, Daniel, the prophets, Jesus, and Paul launched great ministries after extended periods of fasting. Entire nations and cities declared fasts in times of crisis or during times of repentance and soul-searching during ancient times.

Fasting is the Creator's high-powered spiritual tool for receiving a breakthrough in body, soul, and spirit. People in virtually every civilization and culture have an instinctive understanding of the power of fasting and what it can do to clear the mind and the body.

Fasting is a great practice when you feel lethargic or ill. Anyone who has been sick understands that in times of sickness, hunger pangs tend to end. Any attempt to bypass those signals and eat often results in violent regurgitation or other discomfort.

Fast and Be Happy

The Bible describes numerous fasts that varied according to type, length, and purpose. Let's take a closer look:

* The three-day "Esther fast" (see Esther 4:16), considered a "crisis fast," is a total fast from all food and liquids for three days. Many people observe this fast when they face difficult decisions, worries, or spiritual concerns. Due to our poor level of health and the abundance of toxins within our tissues, however, total fasts—meaning abstaining from all food *and* water or liquids—should not be attempted today.
* The ten-day "Daniel fast" is a modified fast with virtually unlimited applications. This fast is named after the biblical Daniel and his Hebrew companions who fasted from rich meats (which possibly could have been unclean meats like pork or shellfish) and wine, choosing to consume "pulse" or

the ripe, edible seeds and produce of a wide range of plants
instead.

* The results were phenomenal as Daniel and his friends out-
performed their contemporaries who supped the usual foods
and wine at the King's table. Daniel and his colleagues continued on this diet for *three years*. (Read the first chapter of
Daniel.)

* You may choose a fast that eliminates sugar, caffeine, carbon-
ated soft drinks, junk foods, pasteurized dairy products, commercial breakfast cereals, or pork products. Such a fast would
be an excellent way to break free from food addictions or
certain eating habits and launch a healthier lifestyle.

* Daniel also completed a very serious 21-day, water-only fast
as well. Make sure you confer with your health professional
before beginning such an extreme fast. Extended water-only
fasts should only be performed under strict supervision of a
licensed physician. Some health conditions make this a risky
choice, which is why it's better to be safe than sorry.

* Moses and Jesus both completed miraculous forty-day total
fasts (without liquids), but I wouldn't recommend under-
taking this type of total fast from food and water—unless
you're expecting a miracle. Serious damage is done to internal organs and body chemistry beyond the three-day point of
dehydration.

* Many people have completed forty-day water and diluted juice
fasts using diluted low-acid fruit or vegetable juices. These
fasts, however, should be undertaken with great care and
under the supervision of a health professional. Doing these
types of fasts repeatedly has been known to trigger permanent
undesirable metabolism changes in the body. In fact, I know
of one man who completed more than fifteen such fasts; he
was formerly slim and trim, but he developed ongoing problems with obesity and blood sugar regulation.

"Take Some Chicken Broth, and Call Me in the Morning!"

The average person feels much better and lives healthier by observing a one-day cleansing fast each week. Many health practitioners are returning to the proven wisdom of selected fasting in the treatment of major toxicities. Some involve "mono fasts" where people eat only one food or fast from a particular food group. Sometimes they recommend that people go on a chicken broth fast, which is another kind of modified fast.

History has proven that the body can heal itself from many serious conditions by fasting, and today the health-care community is beginning to catch on. Even a partial-day fast can be beneficial. This is why I recommend a weekly one-day partial fast from dinner to dinner in my forty-day health program, which is outlined in Chapter 12.

Remember, the body heals while it fasts and undergoes an important regeneration process during our nightly break from activity and eating. That is why our first meal is called breakfast—we are breaking the fast that heals.

Dr. William L. Esser followed the progress of 156 patients at his West Palm Beach retreat center in Florida who agreed to undergo therapeutic fasts of various lengths. He reported on the fasting results of these 156 people who complained of symptoms from thirty-one medically diagnosed diseases, including ulcers, tumors, tuberculosis, sinusitis, pyorrhea, Parkinson's disease, heart disease, cancer, insomnia, gallstones, epilepsy, colitis, hay fever, bronchitis, asthma, and arthritis.

The shortest fast among these 156 patients lasted five days; the longest lasted fifty-five days. Only 20 percent of his patients fasted as long as Dr. Esser recommended, however. The results are as follows:

* 113 completely recovered.
* 31 partially recovered.
* 12 were not helped.
* 92 percent improved or totally recovered

Selected forms of fasting may bring improvement to a number of physical conditions including arthritis, intestinal problems, obesity, and even diabetes.

Finally, keep this thought in mind: If you have a physical condition and are considering a fast, make sure you consult with your health professional first. In general, anyone with diabetes or hypoglycemia should only observe a fast with the approval and ongoing supervision of a health-care provider knowl-edgeable in the management of blood sugar and insulin as related to diabetes. Pregnant or breast-feeding women should not fast at all.

Join the Coated Tongue and Bad Breath Crowd

Observing water-only or liquids-only fasts in today's toxic world may place a considerable burden on the body, but at times the benefits far outweigh the difficulties. What difficulties? Arthur Wallis, author of *God's Chosen Fast: A Spiritual and Practical Guide to Fasting*, outlines a few difficulties:

> The pores of the skin, the mouth, the lungs, the kidneys, the liver and, of course, the bowels are all involved, so the medical experts tell us, in this physical spring-cleaning. The unpleasant taste in the mouth, coated tongue, and bad breath are all part of the process.
>
> There is the familiar "fasting headache," mostly caused by the reac-tion of the body to the sudden cessation of tea and coffee, sugar and other stimulants—a mild "withdrawal" symptom as the body accustoms itself to being without the caffeine drug.... There is also the tendency to sleeplessness, bouts of abdominal discomfort, nau-sea, dizziness, and, of course, weakness....
>
> It is a physical and spiritual medicine, and our usual verdict on such, however well the pharmacist may sugar-coat the pill, is: "Unpleas-ant, but good for you."

Wallis also presents a list of benefits from fasting that include bright eyes, pure breath and skin, and a renewed sense of well-being, adding, "A Christian worker after only a five-day fast declared, 'I feel as though I've got a brand-new stomach.' A digestive weakness he had for years disappeared."

Finally, understand that the most crucial time of any fast is *at the end* when you begin to reacclimatize your cleansed digestive system to foods once again. Do not gorge yourself on breads, meats, or even large amounts of vegetables. Your stomach, which shrank during the fasting process, will stretch out again, but this should happen gradually.

Be sure to break longer fasts with broths and non-acidic liquids such as raw vegetable juices, vegetables, fruits, and raw cultured dairy for the first few meals. Then gradually work your way back to a regular diet over a period of two to four days, depending on the length and extent of your fast.

Roll: Move, Exercise, Get Up, and Do Something!

The advice to "roll" for anyone whose life seems to be going up in flames is simple and easily followed.

First of all, God created us to live, move, work, play, overcome obstacles, and win victories throughout life. He never intended for us to sit around and wait for death. Some confirmed couch potatoes have confidently justified their lackadaisical approach to life by quoting the passage from the King James Bible, "For bodily exercise profiteth little…" (1 Timothy 4:8, KJV).

They conveniently forget that Timothy probably walked everywhere he went and got more exercise in one day than most people today get in a week. Modern translations more accurately paint the picture and remove the lazy boy loophole, saying, "For physical training is of *some value*" (1 Timothy 4:8, NIV, with emphasis added).

What Was It You Were Waiting for Again?

We have a world to explore and make the most of, and we can't do that if our bodies are accumulating fat and our muscles, joints, and internal organs are breaking down. We all need exercise.

Since Richard Simmons released his aerobic videos in the 1980s, the extended-exertion theory of aerobic exercise has ruled supreme in medical and physical fitness circles. This theory maintains that maximum health comes from exercising the cardiovascular system to elevated or maximum stress levels for sustained or unbroken time periods (usually thirty minutes or more). The belief is that this trains or strengthens the cardiovascular system much like a bodybuilder exercises muscles through applied stress to achieve maximum size or strength.

This may be true, but the weakness of this theory comes from its foundation in the flawed "clogged artery/high cholesterol" theories of cardiovascular disease. Lower cholesterol rates have no connection with lower incidences of heart attack or heart disease; it is better to use the genuinely accurate homocysteine levels and oxidative stress as risk factors.

Unfortunately, sustained aerobic exercise has worn out joints and cartilage and inflicted serious chronic sports injuries at rates higher than anyone
predicted. Even worse, aerobically fit people with low cholesterol levels are
dropping dead from heart attacks just as often as those who never exercise
and have terrible cholesterol levels. This may be due to the fact that people
who regularly perform aerobic exercise for long periods of time experience a
weakened immune system. This drop in immunity makes them prime targets
for infections.

We do need exercise for maximum health, but high-stress aerobic exercise
doesn't deliver as promised.

Exercise Should Mirror Real Life

From my research, I am convinced the Creator's prescription for exercise
more closely resembles real-life activities involved in the daily patterns of work
and play.

The longest-lived peoples in human history usually walked everywhere
they went, trailed their animals and herds, hunted wild game on foot, built
rugged shelters, or cultivated fields at an active pace with intermittent periods of rest. They knew nothing about aerobic exercise, treadmills, or CrossFit,
but they were masters at anaerobic exercise—activities that incur an "oxygen
debt" through temporary or briefly sustained exertion.

Current fashion fads aside, we don't need to look as muscular as the people
we see on television or on magazine covers, but anyone can certainly be a lot
healthier with a nutritious diet and moderate exercise. I am not completely
against aerobic exercise, but if your goal is to live a healthier life free of disease
and needless health complications, there are certain exercises that are much
better for your overall health.

Walking

My description of the oldest physical activity of the human race can be
expressed in one word: walking. Even before Eve, Adam was assigned the
task to care for God's garden—a job that could not be done without walking.
Subsequent generations in biblical times demanded even more walking.

A brisk two-mile walk (with long strides and vigorous arm movement)
every day increases enzyme and metabolic activity and may increase calorie
burning for up to twelve hours afterward.

Don't waste time looking for choice parking spots close to your destination—choose a spot far away and walk there. This takes care of two important priorities at once—you get what you came for, and you're getting healthful exercise, too! (And forget the elevators and escalators—take the stairs.) Take a walk on the beach or to the corner store, but don't buy junk food for the return trip! You can even "walk the mall" when the weather doesn't cooperate.

Functional Fitness

Functional fitness is a system of exercise that is truly holistic. Functional fitness utilizes movements that are natural to the body and enhance the health and strength of every muscle. Unlike traditional bodybuilding, functional training focuses on improving the strength of the body's core (the abdominals and lower back), which also houses many of our most important organs.

Functional fitness can be used to achieve great results by people of all walks of life, from the professional athlete who wants to improve performance to the grandmother who wants to climb the stairs to her bedroom more easily. Functional fitness expert Juan Carlos Santana says it best: "One of the main things that the body is intended for is to provide structure and movement. Therefore, functional fitness would be any training that enhances the body's structure and/or movement."

There's no doubt in my mind that functional fitness is the most effective exercise and fitness system available. Functional fitness has been my go-to form of fitness for many years now.

Deep-breathing Exercises

Deep-breathing exercises increase the fat-burning metabolism of your body and boost your brain with a rich dose of oxygen. Deep breathing offers benefits that might make a major difference in your health. Your lungs are larger at the bottom than at the top, but most people in America are "top breathers." We live on the shallow breaths common to the sick and the sleeping.

Learn to breathe from the gut. You know you're breathing from the diaphragm if you can see your stomach move in and out. If the only thing that moves or expands is your chest, then you are still living on a shallow percentage of the divine potential for deep breathing.

Deep breathing literally massages and moves the soft internal organs inside your rib cage, allowing your lymph system to rid itself of collected toxins and to collect even more. Only deep breathing allows you to tap the "bonus power" of your lower lungs.

Newborn babies instinctively deep breathe—watch and learn at the next opportunity. We actually learn how to shallow breathe and rob ourselves of the breath of life. Keep in mind that the way you breathe is important. Singers, stage performers, broadcast announcers, and professional athletes pay great sums to voice coaches and breathing coaches to learn how to breathe, project the voice, and achieve maximum strength through diaphragm breathing.

Here's a quick course to get you started:

1. Sit or lie down and relax.
2. Place a hand your abdomen to see if it expands as you breathe. If only your chest moves with your breaths, you are shallow breathing.
3. Breathe deeply through your mouth, and breathe all the way down to your belly button. Your abdomen (stomach) should rise as you inhale, but not your chest.
4. Hold your breath for a few seconds, and then exhale slowly and fully. Learn to recognize the sounds and sensations of long, slow, deep breaths as your Maker intended. With more practice, you will revert back to the instinctive deep breathing way you began life.

Rebounding

One way to get the exercise you need is by rebounding, which is using a portable mini-trampoline to jump, hop, twist, jog, or step walk in place.

One respected advocate of rebounding uses the devices and rebounding techniques in his rehabilitation program. According to James White, Ph.D., director of research and rehabilitation in the physical education department of the University of California at San Diego (UCSD), "When you jump, jog, and twist on a rebounder device, you can exercise for hours without getting tired. It's great practice for skiing, improves your tennis strokes, and is a good way to burn off calories and lose weight." Dr. White believes it is more effective for fitness and weight loss than cycling, running, or jogging—while producing fewer injuries.

If you're stuck indoors, try some rebounding exercise in which you jump on a mini-trampoline. Rebounding is very good for the lymphatic system, the circulatory system, and the spine while sparing your joints and ligaments.

Even a Little Bit Helps

Because we're much less active than we used to be, even a little exercise goes a long way. An article in Consumer Reports on Health described a study of 13,000 men and women at the Cooper Institute for Aerobics Research in Dallas, Texas. The researchers conducted the eight-year study hoping to prove the value of consistent aerobic exercise, based on how long the volunteers could stand to exercise on a treadmill. The study said this:

> As fitness increased, the death rate fell. But by far, the biggest drop in mortality—60 percent for men, nearly 50 percent for the women—occurred between the most unfit volunteers and those who were just slightly more fit.

Regardless of where you land on the exercise scale, this should make you feel better. Even if you don't exercise at all, or the last time you exercised was on the schoolyard, you can begin to improve your health immediately by starting to exercise now.

I hope this chapter has served as a tune-up, a service-warning light in your health dashboard. Even if you faithfully follow the guidelines and food recommendations of the Maker's Diet, you will need to practice the philosophy of "stop, drop, and roll" on a regular basis.

Don't wait until you smell smoke or your engine sputters and quits. Learn to read your body's symptoms and discern the familiar warning signs. At the first sign of fire or flames burning where they shouldn't be, stop everything to rest, fast, and exercise a little. It doesn't take much to recharge your battery.

Even when you are trying to do everything right, there may be those times when you need some of the Maker's medicine. Fortunately for us, He has supplied them in abundance.

In the rigors of daily life, you may need to take a hot/cold shower, anoint yourself with essential oils, listen to music that soothes the soul, and allow the warmth of a hot bath to soak deep into your aching bones. This may seem like a description for a day at the spa, but it's really just biblical medicine.

≈

11

Biblical Medicine: Herbs, Essential Oils, Hydrotherapy, and Music Therapy

T HE PROPHET EZEKIEL PROVIDED US WITH A FASCINATING, BIBLICAL portrait of divine health when he spoke of healing leaves and refreshing fruit:

> *Along the bank of the river, on this side and that, will grow all kinds of trees used for food; their leaves will not wither, and their fruit will not fail. They will bear fruit every month, because their water flows from the sanctuary. Their fruit will be for food, and their leaves for medicine.*
>
> —EZEKIEL 47:12 (NKJV)

If you were to send someone from our Western civilization to buy medicine today, he will head for the nearest pharmacy. If you were to send someone from East Asia or Central and South America out for medicine, he will likely head for the nearest herb garden or herbal outgrowth in the wild and return with herbs or essentials oils extracted from the herbs of the field.

An herb is defined by Merriam-Webster's Dictionary as a "seed-bearing annual, biennial or perennial that does not develop persistent woody tissue but dies down at the end of a growing season" [unlike a tree, for instance] or "a plant or plant part valued for its medicinal, savory or aromatic qualities." The Maker's herbs were humanity's first medical resource. They remain an important source of healing and nutritional support, although many in our Western culture don't realize it.

According to Rex Russell, M.D., thousands of herbal ingredients have been identified by chemists for their health-promoting qualities, and the pharmaceutical industry is constantly searching for more plant ingredients to isolate and mass distribute in purer forms. "Twenty-five percent of all drugs still come from herbs," Dr. Russell said.

Herbs and spices are incredible sources of antioxidants with antimicrobial and anti-inflammatory properties. According to James Balch, M.D., author of Prescription for Natural Healing, herbs have an important advantage over isolated drugs. The powerful chemicals they contain treat specific health problems while other ingredients in the herbs "balance" those chemicals, making them less toxic while improving their medicinal effectiveness.

We can look to Scripture to see how herbs have been used by people for thousands of years. Medicinal herbalist James A. Duke, Ph.D., former chief of the USDA Medicinal Plant Laboratory and author of Herbs of the Bible: 2000 Years of Plant Medicine, states, "The Bible mentions 128 plants that were part of the everyday life of ancient Israel and of its Mediterranean neighbors." Many of those plants can still be found in Israel today. Dr. David Darom, a botanist, has identified and photographed eighty kinds of plants mentioned in the Bible that are still growing in Israel today.

The Bible often mentions herbs, although it rarely goes into great detail about the use of healing herbs. Herbs were highly valued in biblical times, though, and herb or "vegetable" gardens spawned murder plots and national atrocities. King Ahab's wife, the infamous Jezebel, took matters into her own lethal hands when Naboth refused to sell his vineyard. (The New International and New American versions translate this word as "vegetable garden.") Naboth was wrongfully stoned, and King Ahab suddenly had the vineyard and garden he always wanted. (See 1 Kings 21:2–13.)

Natural herbs promote healing, preserving health, and improving our quality of life. I've listed twenty-one of the top biblical herbs to whet your appetite so you can learn how they can improve your life. Many of these herbs are used as seasonings, some are edible in salads or soups, and some can be used to make teas. I've found it beneficial to incorporate these wonderful substances into your everyday diet.

Twenty-One of the Maker's Most Healing Herbs

Of the fantastic variety of herbs the Creator gave to us, which are constantly being studied for their healthful uses, I consider the following twenty-one herbs to be among the top healing herbs known to man.

1. Aloes

Aloes are mentioned in the Bible when Joseph of Arimathea, a secret follower of Jesus, asked Pilate for permission to bury Jesus following His death by crucifixion. When Joseph received consent, he was accompanied by Nicodemus, who blunted or neutralized the smell of death by bringing a mixture of aloes and myrrh totaling seventy-five pounds, which they used when they wrapped the body of Jesus in strips of linen. (See John 19:39–40.)

Then, in 1492, aloe vera "sailed the ocean blue" with Columbus on his way to discovering America. These days, aloe vera appears in countless American kitchens and bathrooms as front-line treatment for burns and skin irritations.

Aloe vera also purges the stomach and lower intestines when taken internally, but caution should be exercised here. Also, aloe vera aids in the healing of open sores.

Aloes, which come from short-stemmed succulent plants, have anesthetic and antibacterial properties and literally increase blood or lymph flow in small vessels when applied topically. Aloe vera can be used for teenage acne, or you can try heating an aloe vera leaf and applying it directly to abscesses, bruises, skin inflammations, gumboils, or even sprains like the Yucatec Mayans do in Mexico and Belize.

2. Black cumin (Nigella sativa)

This biblical herb, popular in breads and cakes, is used medicinally to purge the body of worms and parasites. An Arab proverb calls black cumin "the medicine for every disease except death."

Black cumin seeds taste hot to the tongue and are sometimes mixed with peppercorns in Europe. The oil of black cumin contains nigellone, which protects guinea pigs from histamine-induced bronchial spasms, which explains its use to relieve the symptoms of asthma, bronchitis, and coughs. The presence of the antitumor sterol, beta sitosterol, lends some credence to its use in folklore to treat abscesses and tumors of the abdomen, eyes, and liver.

3. Black mustard (Brassica nigra)

The Greeks were the first to name this herb that grew wild along the Sea of Galilee. Black mustard seeds contain both a fixed and an essential oil and have been used in plasters and been applied externally to treat numerous conditions such as arthritis and rheumatism.

According to Dr. Duke, research has revealed five compounds in mustard that support cellular structure. Mustard applied to skin surfaces causes blood vessels to enlarge and shed body heat, which explains its use for treating congestion, neuralgia, or muscle spasms. Breathing in steam produced by hot water poured over bruised mustard seeds is also good for colds and headaches.

4. Cinnamon (Cinnamomum verum)

This delightful herb was part of the holy oil used to anoint priests and vessels in the tabernacle of Moses (Exodus 30:22–25). Cinnamon was also mentioned in setting the stage for romance in Proverbs. Ancient Chinese used cinnamon to treat health conditions in China as early as 2700 B.C.

Originally imported from India and Sri Lanka during biblical times, this herb has become one of America's favorite spices because of the way cinnamon calms the stomach. Recent research indicates cinnamon contains antiseptic properties that kill bacteria-causing tooth decay and disease-causing fungi and viruses. Cinnamon may suppress urinary tract infections (UTI) and infestations of Candida.

Dr. Duke reports that USDA researchers discovered that cinnamon reduces the amount of insulin necessary for glucose metabolism in type 2 diabetes. You don't need much: just one-eighth teaspoon of this herb triples insulin efficiency. A warning must be issued about cinnamon oil, which is known as a powerful germicide that may cause vomiting or kidney damage.

5. Coriander (Coriandrum sativum)

In its green form, this herb—also known as cilantro and Chinese parsley—has been used traditionally by those suffering from acid indigestion, neuralgia, rheumatism, and toothaches. History records its use as early as 1550 B.C. for culinary and medicinal purposes.

Coriander was one of the medicines employed by Hippocrates around 400 B.C. There is some research that shows cilantro can support the elimination of harmful metals from the body, including mercury, lead, and cadmium.

Coriander contains twenty natural chemicals possessing antibacterial properties that help control body odor; as mentioned, this essential oil has been used by those dealing with indigestion and excess gas.

6. Cumin (Cuminum cyminum)

Cumin, which has incredible antioxidant properties, was used in biblical times as a medicine and appetite stimulant. This brownish yellow herb has been traditionally used as a remedy for arrhythmia (abnormal heartbeat), asthma, dermatitis, and impotence. The oil of this aromatic seed was used as a disinfectant, perhaps because it's bactericidal and larvicidal and possesses anesthetic properties.

Dr. Duke notes, "My research shows that the spice contains three pain-relieving compounds and seven anti-inflammatory properties. If I had carpal tunnel syndrome, I would add lots of cumin to my curried rice and other spicy dishes."

7. Dandelion (Taraxacum officinale)

One of the candidates for the bitter herbs eaten at Passover, dandelion has been used traditionally as a remedy for cancer, diabetes, hepatitis, osteoporosis, and rheumatism. Contemporary herbalists recommend dandelion almost exclusively as a diuretic for weight loss because this herb provides potassium rather than depleting it as diuretic drugs do.

The green leaves of the dandelion are rich in vitamin C and contain more beta carotene than carrots, and its roots act as a diuretic and purgative useful for supporting kidney and liver function.

8. Dill (Anethum graveolens)

This common ingredient for modern do-it-yourself "picklers" was so historically valued at one time that the ancient Israelites were required to tithe from their supplies. The ancient Greeks and Romans also cultivated dill as a kitchen herb. Dill has been used traditionally as a support for cellular and estrogen deficiency, and research supports dill's three-thousand-year use as a digestive aid and support for excessive intestinal gas.

Dill seed oil inhibits the growth of several bacteria that attach to the digestive tract. As a tea, it soothes the stomach in amazing way, and its oil is so strongly antibacterial that it inhibits organisms such as Bacillus anthracis. Dill contains various phytochemicals that enhance estrogen levels and supports the body's fight against infection, bacteria, and insects.

9. Henna (Lawsonia inermis)

This fragrant herb yields a dark red dye that's used for chemical-free brownish chestnut hair dye formulas today. Widely used in the cosmetics industry, henna can dye just about anything—and will stick around for a long time.

Dr. Duke reports that Egyptian mummies exhumed after three thousand years in a tomb still had traces of henna dye on their nails! Henna contains lawsone, an active antibacterial often used to treat fungal infections of the nails.

10. Fenugreek (Trigonella foenum-graecum)

This herb may be what the Bible calls "leeks." Long considered the "cure-all" treatment for ailments in the Middle East, Dr. Duke reports that fenugreek's bittersweet seeds contain five compounds that appear to promote lower blood sugar levels in the body.

11. Frankincense (Boswellia sacra)

Frankincense, one of the three gifts presented to Jesus by the Magi, was not native to Israel. This "milk" of the frankincense shrub came from sap seeping through cuts made in the plant's bark. Frankincense was also one of the four exclusive components used to make holy incense for the tabernacle of Moses and is still used today by the Roman Catholic Church as well as in a number of expensive perfumes and colognes.

12. Garlic (Allium sativum)

This ancient herb has more going for it than its unmatched flavor in sauces, bread, and meats. Used for centuries as an effective infection fighter, garlic has been used as a painkiller and for the way this herb stimulates the immune system and supports cardiovascular health.

13. Hyssop (Hyssopus officinalis or Origanum syriacum)

This herb, also called marjoram, is harvested from dry places among rocks. A spice, a tonic, and a digestive aid, hyssop was the Bible's "brush of salvation" for spreading the blood of lambs on doorposts to spare the Israelites from the death angel in Egypt. Hyssop was also used in purification ceremonies to cleanse those who came into contact with lepers or corpses. Hyssop stops bleeding (as an astringent) and effectively masks odors; it has been used traditionally to support respiratory function and inflammation as well as a digestive aid.

14. Juniper (Juniperus oxycedrus)

This conifer still grows in Israel and is likely to be the "algum timber" that King Solomon requested of Hiram, king of Tyre, in 2 Chronicles 2:8–9. Juniper yields two forms of cade oil prized for use in men's fragrances, antiseptic soaps, and as a smoked flavor in meats. Cade oil has long been used to treat skin parasites in animals, and it's finding new uses as a treatment for human psoriasis, eczema, and other skin and scalp conditions.

Dr. Duke reports that researchers recently identified certain lignans in juniper that could be used in the production of etoposide, a drug used to support cellular structure. They also found a potent antiviral compound in junipers that can fight various viruses.

15. Milk thistle (Silybum marianum)

This ancient herb native to Samaria and parts of Israel has been used as a liver remedy for two millennia, perhaps because it contains silymarin, a natural compound that supports liver health.

The German government has approved milk thistle seeds and extracts for use in treating chronic liver conditions. Milk thistle, which can be grown in home gardens, has been shown to support blood sugar and insulin levels. Its seeds contain eight anti-inflammatory compounds that aid in healing skin conditions and infections.

16. Mint or horsemint (Mentha longifolia)

Mint or "sweet-scented plants" are mentioned in two Gospels where Jesus scolded the Pharisees for gladly giving a tenth of their garden herb harvest to God while failing to honor Him in far more important matters. (See Matthew 23:23 and Luke 11:42.) The Jewish people enjoyed mint with their spring Passover feasts and placed mint on the floors of their synagogues.

Some species of mint are used to flavor candies, gum, toothpaste, and liqueurs and are also used as digestive aids. Peppermint oil is antiallergenic and is used in aromatherapy to stimulate brain activity.

17. Myrrh (Cistus inanus or Commiphora erythraea)

According to Dr. Duke, there are 135 varieties of myrrh found throughout Africa and Arabia. Myrrh oil was used in the purification of Esther and the other virgin candidates to prepare them to appear before King Xerxes. (See Esther 2:12.)

The aromatic herb was administered both as oils for the exterior and as edible substances for internal cleansing. Persian kings even wore myrrh in their crowns. This expensive, fragrant herb was used to make the holy anointing oil used in the tabernacle of Moses and was one of the gifts given to Jesus Christ by the Magi.

Myrrh was a cure-all treatment in Mesopotamia, Greece, and the Roman Empire. These days, myrrh used in a mouthwash can stop infections, and the herb is an effective treatment for bronchial and vaginal infections.

Myrrh contains a compound called furanosesquiterpenoid, which deactivates a protein in cancer cells that resists chemotherapy, according to researchers at Rutgers University. This compound has proven effective against leukemia, breast cancer, and cancers of the prostate, ovaries, and lungs.

18. Nettle (Urtica dioica)

"Stinging nettles" get their name from the Latin term urtica ("to burn") because the tiny hairs on the leaves cause a burning sensation when touched, similar to bee stings and snakebites. Mentioned in the Book of Job, nettles may contain substances that alleviate arthritis symptoms; they are also rich sources of vitamins A, C, and E as well as many antioxidants.

19. Saffron (Crocus sativus)

This flowering herb served as a condiment, sweet perfume, and coloring agent in biblical times as well as the world's most expensive spice. The reason why: one ounce of saffron requires 4,300 flowers.

Each autumn, saffron flowers are picked in the morning when they first open because the three orange-scarlet stigmas inside the flowers must be taken before the flowers wilt. Saffron dyed the clothes and hands of Jewish spice merchants with a yellow hue in the Middle Ages, so they were often called "saffron merchants."

Saffron yellow was used to mock Jews for centuries, but never so cruelly as in Nazi Germany's requirement that all Jews wear armbands bearing a yellow

Star of David. Saffron was used medically in tinctures for treating gastric and intestinal problems and is considered antispasmodic and is an expectorant, a sedative, or a stimulant in small doses. This herb is also helpful for bladder, kidney, and liver ailments.

20. Spikenard (Nardostachys grandiflora or jatamansi)

A woman of the streets won eternal fame when she humbly anointed Jesus with an alabaster box filled with spikenard, worth a year's wages. The plant was imported from India, and the oils were used in cosmetics and perfumes and medically dispensed as a stimulant.

The spikenard's rhizome, or large root, contains jatamansi, a compound used to combat epilepsy. Infusions are used to treat epilepsy, hysteria, heart palpitations, and chorea. Spikenard oil may support auricular flutter or abnormal heart rhythm, and it acts to depress the central nervous system and relax skeletal and soft tissue muscles.

21. Turmeric (Curcuma longa)

This herb and spice possesses tremendous anti-inflammatory and antioxidant properties. Much of the research conducted on turmeric has been done in India, which shows how this herb may be beneficial as a wound treatment, digestive aid, liver protector, and heart tonic.

Turmeric is a potent spice for cooking and flavor enhancement, and when used in powdered form, it's an antioxidant. This peppery spice is a reliable chemical indicator that changes color when in contact with alkaline and acid substances.

Turmeric's essential oil has been proven to exhibit anti-inflammatory and anti-arthritic qualities. Known as a pain reliever older than aspirin, turmeric rivals the newest exotic painkillers in its ability to relieve aches and pains without upsetting the stomach.

I highly recommend the use of these biblical herbs as an integral part of any healing regimen. Try to add these herbs and spices to your daily diet, or take a nutritional supplement containing oil-based extracts of these life-giving substances.

The Maker's Healing Oils

The Bible mentions at least thirty-three species of essential oils and makes more than one thousand references to their use in:

* maintaining wellness
* acquiring healing
* enhancing spiritual worship
* helping with emotional cleansing
* aiding purification from sin
* setting apart individuals for holy purposes.

These essential oils were inhaled, applied topically, and taken internally. So why are so many missing from our lives today?

Answer: because manufacturers of personal care products have found it much cheaper to produce chemical and synthetic versions.

This is a shame, especially in light of the fact that 70 percent of the books in the Bible mention essential oils, their uses, and/or the plants from which they are derived. We should consider their immense value when we understand the importance, after being mentioned so many times in Scripture, given to them by the Creator. We do know that essential oils have the highest ORAC (oxygen radical absorbance capacity) scores of any substance in the world. The ORAC scale measures the antioxidant powers of foods and other substances.

Four important biblical essential oils greatly outperform the highest-ranking fruits and vegetables in existence. For example, one ounce of clove oil has the antioxidant capacity of 450 pounds of carrots, 120 quarts of blueberries, or 48 gallons of beet juice. Essential oils are composed of very small molecules that can pass through the blood-brain barrier freely or pass through the skin and reach every part of your body in minutes. If you place a drop of cinnamon or peppermint oil on the sole of your foot, you may taste it on your tongue in less than sixty seconds.

The fourteen biblical essential oils I have listed below contain three unique classes of compounds. The first are phenylpropanoids, which are antiviral and anti-bacterial. These phenylpropanoids are able to clean and reprogram "receptor" sites in individual body cells. The second are sesquiterpenes, which possess a variety of healing properties and the ability to reprogram scrambled or damaged DNA coding. And the third and last are monoterpenes, which deliver oxygen directly to cells and possess anti-carcinogenic properties.

Personal Benefits

Perhaps we should consider that the divine instructions for biblical anointing affected the physical realm far more than we formerly believed. You may enjoy significant health benefits by utilizing essential oils for yourself, your family, and your home. I encourage you to anoint yourself with an essential oil and investigate these claims for yourself.

Place a few drops of one of the biblical essential oil blends on your palm, making several clockwise circles with your fingers. Then rub your palms together and cup them over your nose and mouth (but make sure you avoid touching your eyes). Deeply inhale the aromatic vapors, then run your fingers and palms through your hair. It won't make your hair "oily," but it will transform the way you feel.

Another great way to use essential oils is to put five to ten drops into a warm bath. That is a true healing treat. You can also rub a few drops of these oils into the soles of your feet. You can even gain benefit from inhaling directly from the bottle. If you have small children, try applying essential oils to their stuffed animals or to the inside of their pillowcases each night.

The following list is fourteen of the most useful essential oils with a brief description of their positive effects on the body.

1. Myrrh (Commiphora myrrha)

In days of old, pregnant mothers anointed themselves with myrrh for protection against infectious diseases and to elevate feelings of well-being. Myrrh was also used in ancient times for skin conditions, oral hygiene, embalming, and as an insect repellent. In modern times, myrrh is used to balance the thyroid and endocrine system, support the immune system, heal fungal and viral infections, and enhance emotional well-being.

2. Frankincense (Boswellia carteri)

In biblical times, frankincense was used as a holy anointing oil to enhance meditation, for embalming, and in perfume. Frankincense was used to anoint the newborn sons of kings and priests, which may have been why this fragrant oil was brought to baby Jesus. Today, frankincense is used to help maintain normal cellular regeneration, to stimulate the body's immune system, and as an aid for people suffering from cancer, depression, allergies, headache, herpes, bronchitis, and brain damage resulting from head injuries.

3. Cedarwood (Cedrus libani)

Cedarwood was used traditionally in ritual cleansing after touching a dead body, non-kosher animals like pigs, or anything else considered biblically unclean, such as the bedding of someone who had died. Cedarwood was also used in the cleansing of leprosy and the cleansing of evil spirits. It has been used by cultures around the world for embalming, medicine, disinfecting, personal hygiene, and skin problems.

Today cedarwood is used as an insect repellant, as a hair loss treatment, and for tuberculosis, bronchitis, gonorrhea, and skin disorders (such as acne or psoriasis). Cedarwood has the highest concentration of sesquiterpenes, which can enhance cellular oxygen.

4. Cinnamon (Cinnamomum verum)

Cinnamon and cassia are actually two species of the genus Cinnamomum and have similar fragrances. Both are very effective anti-bacterial and antiviral agents that God provided to protect the Israelites from disease. They support the human immune system in the battle against influenza and cold viruses, and all you have to do is simply inhale them or put them on the soles of your feet. (Caution: Do not apply these powerful oils to sensitive areas of the body because they may be slightly caustic and irritating in these areas. If irritation occurs, apply vegetable oil immediately to cool off the skin.)

5. Cassia (Cinnamomum cassia)

Cassia was an ingredient in Moses' holy anointing oil. Cassia, a cousin of cinnamon, is a potent immune system enhancer.

6. Calamus (Acorus calamus)

This ancient essential oil is rich in phenylpropanoids and is usually used in combination with other essential oils. Calamus was used in holy anointing oil and incense and for perfumes. Known as an aromatic stimulant and tonic for the digestive system, today calamus is used to relax muscles, relieve inflammation, support the respiratory system, and clear kidney congestion after intoxication. This useful essential oil can be taken orally, inhaled as incense, or applied topically over the abdomen.

7. Galbanum (Ferula gummosa)

Historically, galbanum was used as holy anointing oil, perfume, and in various medicines. Today, galbanum is used to treat acne, asthma, coughs, indigestion, muscle aches and pains, wrinkles, and wounds as well as to balance emotions.

8. Onycha (Styrax benzoin)

This essential oil comes from tree resin and is the most viscous of all essential oils. Onycha, which has a characteristic vanilla-like fragrance, has been used as a perfume and is blended into anointing oils and used to heal skin wounds.

Today, this comfortable, soothing, and uplifting essential oil is used to stimulate renal output, treat colic, gas, and constipation, and soothe skin irritations and wounds. Onycha may help control blood sugar levels and can be inhaled for sinusitis, bronchitis, colds, coughs, and sore throats.

9. Spikenard (Nardostachys jatamansi)

In biblical times, spikenard was used as a perfume, medicine, mood enhancer, and preparation for burial. Modern science has shown spikenard to relieve allergies, migraines, and nausea. Spikenard supports the cardiovascular system and calms the emotions.

10. Hyssop (Hyssopus officinalis)

As a principal cleanser in biblical times, hyssop was used in many purification rituals and to drive away evil spirits. Modern science has shown that hyssop can be used to relieve anxiety, arthritis, asthma, respiratory infections, parasites, fungal infections, colds, flu, and wound healing. Hyssop metabolizes fat, increases perspiration, and can aid the body's detoxification of harmful chemicals. Hyssop can provide help to balance emotions.

11. Sandalwood (Santalum album)

Used by the ancients for assistance in meditation, sandalwood is also an aphrodisiac and was used in embalming. Sandalwood contains sesquiterpenes that deprogram misinformation and carry oxygen at the cellular level.

This essential oil can be used in skin care, enhance sleep quality, support the female reproductive and endocrine systems, and provide relief in urinary tract infections.

12. Myrtle (Myrtus communis)

Myrtle was used in various ceremonies in biblical times that involved purification from ritual uncleanness. Today, myrtle can be used to balance hormones, soothe the respiratory system, battle colds and flu, and treat asthma, bronchitis, coughs, and skin conditions, including acne, psoriasis, and blemishes.

13. Cypress (Cupressus sempervirens)

Ancient healers used this essential oil to treat arthritis, laryngitis, swollen scar tissue, and cramps. Today, cypress is used to support the cardiovascular system and promote emotional well-being in times of loss or stress. Cypress also promotes the production of white blood cells and boosts natural defenses. When used topically, cypress is generally massaged along the spine, in the armpits, on the feet, and over the heart and chest.

14. Rose of Sharon (Cistus ladanifer)

Used historically as a perfume and to elevate mood, Rose of Sharon is used today as an antiseptic, as an immune enhancer, and for calming the nerves.

I highly recommend the use of biblical essential oils on a daily basis. Inhaled directly or used in therapeutic baths, these oils can make a subtle but powerful difference in our lives.

The Maker's Hydrotherapy

Is it any wonder that water helps heal us when a large percentage of our bodies are composed of water?

Men and women have found refreshment and healing in water since the beginning of human history. The Greeks and Romans built elaborate baths that are still standing, and in modern times, an American president plagued by polio, Franklin D. Roosevelt, made many pilgrimages to natural mineral baths in Hot Springs, Arkansas, seeking healing for his polio and aching joints. Hydrotherapy, or water healing, is simple and inexpensive in its various forms:

* Bathe by immersion when you want to soak your sore body in a bath. Simply immerse yourself for twenty minutes or so in 95-degree water to soothe nerves, relax muscles, and ease bladder and urinary problems. Add healing herbs, salts, or essential oils increases the effectiveness of the bath.

* Showers often best meet the needs of sore shoulders, upper back, and necks.

* Sitz baths are simply shallow baths deep enough to immerse the bottom and hips (and ease the various physical ailments and pains found in those areas).

* Bathe your extremities—the feet and hands—in one or two buckets or containers large enough to hold them.

There are many ways to use hydrotherapy for the health of your body. Here are just a few:

* Warm up cold feet with a fifteen-minute bath in hot water. For tired feet, go with a cold foot bath.

* For aching or arthritic feet or hands, use two buckets or containers of water, one with hot water and the other with cold. Alternate your feet or hands between the hot bath (sixty seconds) and the cold bath (twenty seconds) for a total of twenty minutes.

* The most effective way to get your blood flowing and to stimulate circulation is to take a shower and alternate between hot and cold water for a minimum period of fifteen minutes (one minute hot followed by one minute cold).

You should make the water as hot as you can handle without burning your skin and as cold as you can handle it without pain. Alternate between hot and cold at least seven times during this period. If one area in particular is sore, then make sure the water is hitting that area directly, if possible.

The Maker's Music Therapy

Two biblical examples that illustrate the virtually untapped power of music stand out to me:

- When King Saul fell victim to an evil spirit, all it took was David playing his harp to bring deliverance and sweet relief. (See 1 Samuel 16:23.)
- When the Israelites encircled impregnable Jericho and blew their trumpets and shouted as commanded by God, the walls came tumbling down "without a shot." (See Joshua 6.)

Music therapy as a healing art is making great inroads in the treatment or rehabilitation of patients battling with autism, Alzheimer's, and Parkinson's disease. Beautiful music seems to exhibit a unique property of organizing or reorganizing cerebral function that has been damaged.

Music is a gift from God that possesses healing and delivering powers, so we should use this gift wisely. The best proof of the power of music is your own heart. How many times have you been emotionally and spiritually moved by music?

King Saul knew enough to call for the minstrel David when the "blues" set in. You should prepare lists of your favorite music, and then play the music often, especially when you're down. Feel the music lift your spirits. Certain types of music, particularly what we call "classical" music and cultural music, can bring about great health benefits. A good time to listen to music is while exercising, which can be very inspiring. Many professional tennis players walk out onto the court with headphones on prior to their matches, listening to music that puts them in the right frame of mind.

Listening to worship music is the best. If you feel overwhelmed by the stresses of the day, I recommend that you listen to your favorite worship music and join in singing the choruses. In my experience, worship and music are virtually indivisible.

Of course, worship cannot be limited to music, but it can certainly play a major role in its expression. Consider these words of wisdom by Bishop Joseph Garlington, a noted African-American spiritual leader, musician, and author:

Worship is like breathing: You were created to do it all the time. It's a lifestyle. When everything imaginable comes against you, worship God. When things finally go your way, worship Him. (Of course, it's easier to worship in the good times.)

Nothing else will be as creative as worship, because you are doing more than expressing faith in the sovereign God. You are creating an atmosphere in your own heart and circumstances that releases faith and enables you to say, "My God is in control of this."

I encourage you to tap into the power of the Maker's music and allow the soaring melodies to drain away stress, build up your soul, and enhance your health. The right music at the right time can calm you, excite you, awaken you, or put you to sleep. Music is a divine tool from the loving hand of God to make everyday life a little healthier.

Moving Forward

We would think it foolish for someone to squander a free membership to an exclusive health spa or exclusive golf country club. Yet, how often do we take the time to partake of God's bounty of healing herbs, essential oils, the relaxation of a soothing hot bath, and listening to soothing and inspirational music?

If you sense it's time for a significant change in your life, then it will most likely happen with a clear-cut decision and a period of commitment. Looking back through the prism of time, God has typically used the time period of forty days to accomplish significant life events.

If you are serious about making a break from the past and starting over again in your quest for maximum health, strength, and vitality, then I welcome you to a forty-day, life-changing experience known as the Maker's Diet.

I'll outline the three-phase program in my next chapter.

≈

12

The Maker's Diet: Your 40-Day Health Experience

A S YOU'VE PROBABLY NOTICED, DIETS AND HEALTH FADS LITTER THE landscape of American culture, but the Maker's original plan for your optimal health and wellness is no fad. The Maker's Diet is at once ancient and new, timely yet timeless. Best of all, *it works!* And the Maker's Diet has been changing lives for well more than ten years, so there's a track record.

Unlike other diets or health programs, the Maker's Diet is designed to improve the four pillars of health—physical, spiritual, mental, and emotional.

Now we're in the final stretch, the place where the Maker's Diet can become a reality and produce a richer life for you. When I originally put this plan together, I felt compelled to develop a scientifically sound, real-life plan that you can live with. My goal is to present the principles of this healing protocol as clearly as possible.

In case you're wondering, forty days is by design. Many times in the Bible when God wanted to trigger a significant "turnaround" on Earth, He instituted a forty-day plan. You can see this demonstrated in the lives of Noah, Moses, Elijah, Ezekiel, and Jesus in Genesis 7:4, Exodus 24:18, 1 Kings 19:8, Ezekiel 4:6, Matthew 4:2, and Acts 1:3.

If you're ready for your significant "turnaround" to restore optimal health to your body—physically, spiritually, mentally, and emotionally—then this simple and doable forty-day investment will pay a lifetime of dividends for you and for those you love. The Maker's Diet 40-Day Health Experience incorporates the same biblical dietary and lifestyle principles that saved my life.

In addition, as a result of my years of research and experience with those who followed the Maker's Diet, I estimate that it's at least ten times as effective as the early version of this program that I used to regain my health and break free from the bondage of disease.

With this revision of *The Maker's Diet*, I have been off all medications for nearly twenty-five years and call myself extremely healthy. After suffering the ravages of continuous exposure to powerful medications during my health challenges, I've completely recovered. My weight of 195 pounds is normal for someone who is six feet, one inch tall, and I live a full, active life, especially when I'm at the family ranch in southern Missouri.

I am still awed by how much my life has changed, considering that I wondered at one time if I would live long enough to see my twenty-first birthday. If an injection, pill, or experimental therapy could have freed me from my painful diseases at the time, I would have paid any amount of money to get it, but God definitely healed me in a natural, practical way through the Maker's Diet.

My mother says it best: I was healed as I feasted on the Word of God and applied His principles—including dietary—to my life. Believe me, these principles of divine health are completely reproducible in your life, too.

Experience Forty Days That Will Change Your Life

Now it is your opportunity to experience the first forty days of the rest of your life—forty days that will change your life forever. The Maker's Diet 40-Day Health Experience is divided into three two-week phases. These three phases are easy to follow, and each features foods that are extremely healthy and delicious.

This plan is designed for results; your success depends significantly on your diligence in following the plan. Every effort has been made to keep the recipes in Appendix A simple and the ingredients widely available. You may experience moments of discouragement when dealing with a new recipe or when facing a week without your favorite junk food or dessert, but it's well worth it to persevere through those times—your future health depends on it.

Keep in mind that the Maker's Diet 40-Day Health Experience is designed to attack the three i's—insulin, infection, and inflammation:

* by balancing *insulin,* you can improve physical, mental, and emotional health, and in turn you balance blood sugar, sharpening concentration and enhancing mood
* by reducing *infection,* you can lessen the toxic burden placed on your body by your daily contact with germs
* by lessening *inflammation,* you can reduce aches and pains and decrease risk factors for such diseases as heart disease and cancer

By attacking these three i's, you can improve appearance and enhance energy, and you can begin to reverse the process of accelerated aging and live life the way you were meant to live it.

Here are some helpful tips to make your 40-Day Health Experience a successful one:

1. Expect to feel changes in your body. When you begin Phase One and avoid consuming certain foods and chemicals that you were addicted to (such as sugar, artificial sweeteners, caffeine, preservatives), you may experience temporary withdrawal symptoms such as headaches, flu-like symptoms, increased carbohydrate cravings, less energy, mood swings, or even temporary changes in bowel habits.

This may also happen due to the increased cleansing of toxins from the body. This "detox reaction," as it is sometimes called, is an indication that the program is working and is usually short lived. Make sure to increase your water intake, and if your body is telling you to rest, then do so.

2. If you mess up and go off the program, do not beat yourself up. You are only one meal away from success. No one is perfect. If you're put in a situation where you must eat foods not recommended on a particular phase of the program (and you better have a really good excuse), it's better to consume all of these "forbidden" foods in a one-hour time period rather than several hours or the entire day. Consuming high-carbohydrate or high-calorie foods within a one-hour time period will minimize the amount of insulin your body can produce or overproduce; this will minimize the amount of fat you will store and limit the damage that will be done.

3.   Make time for fun. I recommend at least one day per week to be a fun day. Don't do anything that resembles work. If you can plan your fun day outside, that is even better because breathing fresh air is very healthy.

4.   Get out in the sun. It is important to spend time in the sun. Exposure to sunlight can be very beneficial for your health and can aid in the balance of hormones, enhance mood, and help to build strong bones.

5.   Take time to chew your food. Digestion of carbohydrate foods begins in the mouth. When you eat starchy, high-carbohydrate foods, it is of the utmost importance to chew each mouthful of food twenty to thirty times. That may seem like quite a chore, but this practice will benefit you immensely. Chewing your food not only aids in digestion, but also the action of chewing can stimulate the body to produce certain chemical hormones that enhance mood as well.

6.   Don't eat when you're angry, sad, scared, or anxious. These emotions all shut down digestion. When you are emotionally out of balance, it is better not to eat at all. I mentioned earlier that when you eat sugar, your immune system can be depressed for up to six hours. You also learned that when you're angry, your immune system can be depressed for up to six hours. So if you go and eat a doughnut while you're angry, half of your day is ruined!

The Three Phases

You will also see that there are three phases to the Maker's Diet. Here are some guidelines to determine what phase you should start on.

If you are significantly overweight or obese, or if you have health problems, I recommend you start on Phase One.

If you are extremely healthy and want to stay that way, or even improve your health, you may start on Phase Three. Even if you start on Phase Three, I believe it will be the healthiest program you have ever been on. I believe it is a good idea, however, for everyone to start on Phase One for at least a few days to reset your metabolism and attack the three i's (insulin, infection, and inflammation).

Here's another tip: Tackle your 40-day Health Experience with a friend or a whole group of friends. Ask around to see if anyone is interested, because it will take determination on your part. Remind yourself that achieving your dream of superb health is a worthwhile goal.

I designed each phase of the Maker's Diet to produce noticeable results, but not through dangerous, quick-weight-loss gimmicks that cause you to gain more weight after the program than you lose while going through it. The all-important third phase shows you how to continue on the path that leads to health for life!

So, I have done my part. Now it's your turn as you begin the Maker's Diet 40-Day Health Experience.

The Maker's Diet

Phase One: Days 1–14

A S WITH VIRTUALLY ANY IMPORTANT TASK OR ENDEAVOR, THE WAY YOU start significantly affects the results you enjoy at the finish.

Phase One of the Maker's Diet is designed to stabilize insulin and blood sugar, reduce inflammation, reduce infection, enhance digestion, and help balance the hormones in your body. This should help you better manage your weight in a healthy manner and significantly improve your overall health.

Best of all, the components of Phase One should greatly reduce your risk of incurring disease. It effectively helps your body reduce insulin sensitivity and balance the omega-3/omega-6 ratio that is so vital to balance levels of inflammation and enhance the health of your immune system, which will reduce chances of infection.

Temporary Food Limitations

After reading through this forty-day program, you will notice that Phase One restricts disaccharide-rich carbohydrate foods such as grains, pastas, breads, sugar, potatoes, corn, beans, and legumes. While it's true that the people of the Bible consumed a diet that contained liberal amounts of grains and other carbohydrate foods, they were higher-quality, lesser-processed carbohydrates and therefore much easier to digest. And because they ate smaller quantities of food (some believe as much as six times less food than we do), their typical diet was close to a modern lower-carbohydrate diet.

Also, these people would have eaten extremely healthy diets since birth, so they weren't hampered by increased insulin sensitivity, endocrine imbalances (including thyroid problems), infection, inflammation, and digestive problems common to people who have been reared with the standard American diet (SAD).

Because Phase One is designed to correct these harmful imbalances, it must temporarily limit even healthy foods such as fruits, whole grains, and honey while allowing for the liberal consumption of protein foods, vegetables, and healthy oils.

The Prayer Factor

The Maker's Diet 40-day Health Experience begins and ends each day with prayers of thanksgiving, prayers for healing, and prayers of petition.

As we discussed, it has now been scientifically proven that prayer works. Try repeating these prayers daily to experience how the God of the ages will work a miracle in your life. I've developed these prayers from many different biblical passages. Even if you have never prayed before, God promises that His Word will never return void (empty), but it will prosper in the thing for which He sends it (Isaiah 55:11).

We can trust God's promises. The following prayers can serve as guidelines for you.

A Morning Prayer for Healing

> Father God, I thank You for creating me in Your image. I praise
> You that I am fearfully and wonderfully made. I confess that You
> are the God that heals, my Great Physician. I ask You to heal my
> body from the top of my head to the soles of my feet. I pray that
> You would regenerate every bone, joint, tendon, ligament, tissue,
> organ, and cell of my body. This is the day that the Lord has made;
> I will rejoice and be glad in it.

An Evening Prayer for Restoration

> Father God, I thank You for sustaining me today. I thank You
> that You are made perfect in my weakness. Your grace is sufficient
> for me. I thank You that Your steadfast love never ceases and
> Your mercies are new every morning. You say in Your Word
> that mourning may come for a night, but the new day will bring

gladness. Bless me with a healing night's sleep. Restore unto me the joy of my salvation. Help me to stay on the path that leads to life.

PHASE ONE: FOODS TO ENJOY

Meat (grass-fed/organic is best)

* Beef
* Veal
* Lamb
* Buffalo
* Venison
* Elk
* Goat
* Meat bone soup/stock
* Liver and heart (must be organic)
* Beef or buffalo sausage or hot dogs (no pork casing—organic and nitrite/nitrate-free is best) (Use sparingly in Phase One.)

Fish (wild freshwater/ocean-caught fish is best; make sure the fish have fins and scales)

* Salmon
* Halibut
* Tuna
* Cod
* Scrod
* Grouper
* Haddock
* Mahi mahi
* Pompano
* Wahoo
* Trout
* Tilapia
* Orange roughy
* Sea bass
* Snapper

- Mackerel
- Herring
- Sole
- Whitefish
- Fish bone soup/stock
- Salmon (canned in spring water)
- Tuna (canned in spring water)
- Sardines (canned in water or olive oil only)

Poultry (pastured/organic is best)

- Chicken
- Cornish game hen
- Guinea fowl
- Turkey
- Duck
- Poultry bone soup/stock
- Chicken or turkey bacon (no pork casing—organic and nitrite/nitrate-free is best)
- Chicken or turkey sausage or hot dogs (no pork casing—organic and nitrite/nitrate-free is best) (Use sparingly in Phase One.)
- Liver and heart (must be organic)

Eggs (high omega-3/DHA is best)

- Chicken eggs (whole with yolk)
- Duck eggs (whole with yolk)

Dairy

- Goat's milk yogurt (plain)
- Homemade kefir from goat's milk
- Soft goat's milk cheese
- Goat's milk hard cheese
- Sheep's milk hard cheeses

Fats and oils (organic is best)

* Oil, butter (ghee)
* Goat's milk butter
* Avocado
* Cow's milk butter, organic
* Extra-virgin coconut oil (best for cooking)
* Extra-virgin olive oil (not best for cooking)
* Flaxseed oil (not for cooking)
* Hempseed oil (not for cooking)
* Goat's milk butter (not for cooking)
* Raw cow's milk butter, grass-fed (not for cooking)
* Expeller-pressed sesame oil
* Coconut milk/cream (canned)

Vegetables (organic fresh or frozen is best)

* Broccoli
* Squash (winter or summer)
* Asparagus
* Beets
* Cauliflower
* Brussels sprouts
* Cabbage
* Carrots
* Celery
* Cucumber
* Eggplant
* Pumpkin
* Garlic
* Onion
* Okra
* Lettuce (leaf of all kinds)
* Spinach
* Mushrooms
* Peas

- Peppers
- String beans
- Tomatoes
- Artichoke (French, not Jerusalem)
- Leafy greens (kale, collard, broccoli rabe, mustard greens, etc.)
- Raw leafy greens (endive, escarole, radicchio, arugula, frisée, etc.)
- Sprouts (broccoli, sunflower, pea shoots, radishes, etc.)
- Sea vegetables (kelp, dulse, nori, kombu, hijiki)
- Raw, fermented vegetables (lacto-fermented only, no vinegar)

Beans and legumes (soaked or fermented is best)

- Small amounts of fermented soybean paste (miso) as a broth
- Lentils

Nuts and seeds (organic, raw, or soaked is best)

- Almonds (raw)
- Pumpkin seeds (raw)
- Hempseed (raw)
- Flaxseed (raw and ground)
- Sunflower seeds (raw)
- Almond butter (raw)
- Hempseed butter (raw)
- Sunflower butter (raw)
- Pumpkin seed butter (raw)
- Tahini, sesame butter (raw)

Condiments, spices, seasonings (organic is best)

- Salsa (fresh or canned)
- Tomato sauce (no added sugar)
- Guacamole (fresh)
- Apple cider vinegar
- Celtic sea salt
- Mustard

- Herbamare seasoning
- Omega-3 mayonnaise
- Umeboshi paste
- Soy sauce (wheat free), tamari
- Raw salad dressings and marinades
- Herbs and spices (no added stabilizers)
- Pickled ginger (preservative and color-free)
- Wasabe (preservative and color-free)
- Organic flavoring extracts (alcohol-based, no sugar added), i.e., vanilla, almond, etc.

Fruits (organic fresh or frozen is best)

- Blueberries
- Strawberries
- Blackberries
- Raspberries
- Cherries
- Grapefruit
- Lemon
- Lime

Beverages

- Purified, nonchlorinated water
- Natural sparkling water, no carbonation added (i.e., Perrier)
- Herbal teas (preferably organic)—unsweetened or with a small amount of honey or Stevia
- Raw vegetable juice (beet or carrot juice—maximum 25 percent of total)
- Lacto-fermented beverages
- Certified organic coffee—buy whole beans, freeze them, and grind yourself when desired; flavor only with organic cream and a small amount of honey.

Sweeteners

* Unheated, raw honey in very small amounts (1 Tbsp. per day maximum)

Miscellaneous

* Goat's milk protein powder

PHASE ONE: FOODS TO AVOID

Meat

* Pork
* Ham
* Bacon
* Sausage (pork)
* Veggie burgers
* Imitation meat products (soy)
* Ostrich
* Emu

Fish and seafood

* Fried, breaded fish
* Catfish
* Eel
* Squid
* Shark
* Avoid *all* shellfish, including crab, clams, oyster, mussels, lobster, shrimp, scallops, and crawfish.

Poultry

* Fried, breaded chicken

Luncheon meat

* Turkey
* Roast beef

* Ham
* Corned beef

Eggs

* Imitation eggs (such as Egg Beaters)

Dairy

* Soy milk
* Rice milk
* Almond milk
* Avoid all dairy products other than those listed in "Foods to Enjoy."

Fats and oils

* Lard
* Margarine
* Shortening
* Soy oil
* Safflower oil
* Canola oil
* Sunflower oil
* Corn oil
* Cottonseed oil
* Any partially hydrogenated oil

Vegetables

* Corn
* Sweet potato
* White potato

Beans and legumes

* Soy beans
* Tofu
* Black beans
* Kidney beans

* Navy beans
* White beans
* Garbanzo beans
* Lima beans

Nuts and seeds

* Honey-roasted nuts
* Walnuts
* Macadamia nuts
* Pecans
* Hazelnuts
* Brazil nuts
* Peanuts
* Peanut butter
* Cashews
* Nuts or seeds dry or roasted in oil

Condiments, spices, seasonings

* All spices that contain added sugar
* Commercial ketchup with sugar
* Commercial barbecue sauce with sugar

Fruits

* Avoid all fruits except berries, grapefruit, limes, and lemons. This includes apples, bananas, apricots, grapes, melon, peaches, oranges, pears, dried fruit, and canned fruit.

Beverages

* Alcoholic beverages of any kind
* Fruit juices
* Sodas
* Chlorinated tap water
* Pre-ground commercial coffee

Grains and Starchy Carbohydrates

* Avoid *all* grains and starchy foods, including bread, pasta, cereal, rice, oatmeal, pastries, and baked goods.

Sweeteners

* Sugar
* Maple syrup
* Heated honey
* Fructose or corn syrup
* All artificial sweeteners, including aspartame, sucralose, Acesulfame K
* Sugar alcohol, including sorbitol and xylitol

Miscellaneous

* Milk or whey protein powder from cow's milk
* Soy protein powder
* Rice protein powder

YOUR DAILY REGIMEN

I have detailed for you a daily regimen for each phase of the protocol and given you sample menus for several days of each two-week phase. Always refer to the "Foods to Enjoy" for the phase in which you are participating in order to create your own healthy, delicious meals with a wide variety of natural, healing foods and beverages.

And be sure to enjoy the wonderful recipes included in Appendix A.

You will notice the designations basic, intermediate, or advanced by each component of the daily regimen. Whether you follow the basic, intermediate, or advanced recommendations will depend on your state of health, available time, and budgetary allowances. Your results from this program will depend on your commitment level and discipline.

"Partial-Fast" Days

I have recommended a partial fast one day per week in each phase. (I recommend Thursday as it is much more difficult to fast during the weekend.)

On the partial-fast days you will not be eating breakfast or lunch. You should still consume your cleansing drink and other supplements. This partial-fast day allows the body to cleanse and rebuild.

Make sure to consume lots of fluids during your partial-fast day, especially raw vegetable juices and pure water. To gain maximum spiritual benefit from your partial-fast days, I recommend praying each time you experience hunger.

Remember to follow the daily regimen diligently in order to reap the greatest results. You may want to copy some of these pages and keep record of your progress by checking the boxes when you have completed each part of the daily regimen.

DAILY REGIMEN FOR PHASE ONE: DAYS 1–14

Morning hygiene

Aromatherapy A.M. (Advanced). Use three drops of a biblical aromatherapeutic blend in the palm of your hand. Rub your hands together, cup them in front of your face, and gently inhale through your nose three or four times. You may then rub the remaining oil into your scalp or into the soles of your feet.

Morning cleansing drink (intermediate)

Mix 2 tablespoons of a whole-food fiber blend and 1–2 tablespoons or 5 caplets of a green superfood blend in 8 to 12 ounces of purified water or diluted vegetable juice. Shake vigorously and drink immediately.

Morning tune-up

Recite morning prayer.

Exercise ten to fifteen minutes. Choose from functional fitness, jumping on a rebounder, performing breathing exercise, or going for a walk around the neighborhood.

Listen to music that uplifts and energizes while you exercise.

Breakfast

See the sample breakfast menus in this 40-Day Plan or check out the recipes in Appendix A.

Breakfast supplements (Basic)

Whole-food multivitamin, 2–3 caplets.

PHASE ONE

Lunch

See the sample lunch menus in this 40-Day Plan or check out the recipes in Appendix A.

Lunch supplements (Basic)

Whole-food multivitamin, 2–3 caplets.

Afternoon cleansing drink (Intermediate)

Mix 2 tablespoons of a whole-food fiber blend and 1–2 tablespoons or 5 caplets of a green superfood blend in 8 to 12 ounces purified water or diluted vegetable juice. Shake vigorously and drink immediately.

Dinner

See the sample dinner menus in this 40-Day Plan or check out the recipes in Appendix A

Dinner supplements (Basic)

Whole-food multivitamin, 2–3 caplets.

Cod liver oil (basic): 1 teaspoon to 1 tablespoon based on sun exposure. If you receive more than two hours of direct sunlight per week, you may take 1–2 teaspoons. If you receive less than two hours of direct sunlight per week, you may take 1 tablespoon.

Evening snack

See sample snack menus in this 40-Day Plan or check out the recipes in Appendix A

Evening wind-down

Recite evening prayer.

Exercise ten to fifteen minutes. Choose from functional fitness, jumping on a rebounder, performing breathing exercise, or going on a walk around the neighborhood.

Listen to music that uplifts and energizes while you exercise.

Aromatherapy P.M. (Advanced) Use three drops of a biblical aromatherapeutic blend in the palm of your hand. Rub your hands together, cup them in front of your face, and gently inhale through your nose three or four times. You may then rub the remaining oil into your scalp or into the soles of your feet.

In bed before 10:30

PHASE ONE

SAMPLE MENUS FOR PHASE ONE

Day 1

Breakfast
Fried eggs (prepared any way you desire: over-easy, medium, or well done. Fry in extra-virgin coconut oil or butter.)
Stir-fried veggies

Lunch
Tuna Salad
Raw carrots and celery

Dinner
French-style London Broil
Green salad

Evening snack
1/2 cup strawberries with 1 ounce of raw goat's milk cheese

Day 2

Breakfast
Vegetable Frittata

Lunch
Coconut Milk Soup

Dinner
Wild Alaskan Salmon with Pecan Pesto
Green salad
Cultured vegetables

Evening snack
Carrot, celery, and raw almond butter

Day 3

Breakfast
Onion, Pepper, and Goat Cheese Omelet
Avocado slices with seasoning

Lunch
Oriental Red Meat Salad

Dinner
Coconut Milk Soup

Easy Broiled Halibut

Green salad

Evening snack
Goat's milk yogurt, raw honey, vanilla, and blueberries

Day 4

Breakfast
None (partial-fast day)

Lunch
None (partial-fast day)

Dinner
Cultured veggies

Green salad

Tuna Steaks, Oriental Style

Evening snack
None (partial-fast day)

PHASE ONE

The Maker's Diet

Phase Two: Days 15–28

CONGRATULATIONS! YOU FINISHED PHASE ONE, THE MOST DIFFICULT part of the Maker's Diet 40-Day Health Experience. I'm sure it was a tough two weeks, but I trust you are convinced it was well worth it.

You should feel much better already. If your goal is to lose unwanted pounds and inches, you are probably feeling pretty good right about now. If it's more energy you desire, you are probably surprised by the surge of new energy you are now feeling. Your digestion has improved, your energy levels have increased, your skin looks better, and your cravings are under control. Let me assure you that you are well on your road to optimal health!

What to Expect

As a result of the healing process that has begun, Phase Two introduces (or reintroduces) a greater variety of foods into your daily diet, including fruit, nuts, and seeds. In Phase Two, you may continue to enjoy all of the foods from the "Foods to Enjoy" list in Phase One while adding the new foods listed for Phase Two.

You will continue to lose excess weight, though many people lose weight at a slower pace during this phase. The health goal at this point may not be to achieve dramatic weight loss, but to continue to move toward your ideal weight as you enjoy greater benefits of enhanced health.

Be encouraged. The Maker's Diet 40-Day Health Experience helps you return to your optimal health levels by restoring your immune system, balancing blood sugar, and creating healthy eating habits that will, hopefully, last a lifetime.

PHASE TWO

Remember, you are not trying to squeeze yourself into someone's fanciful idea about how everyone should look. By returning to "the Manufacturer's specifications," your body will naturally return to its ideal weight, shape, and strength levels—all without dangerous side effects.

By the end of Phase Two, you should really be feeling good about yourself because you will have accomplished what very few people even dare to try: you changed your life for the better!

PHASE TWO

PHASE TWO: NEW FOODS TO ENJOY

Feel free to add the following new foods for Phase Two and enjoy them along with the "Foods to Enjoy" from Phase One.

Meat (grass-fed/organic is best)

- All meats listed in Phase One

Fish (wild freshwater/ocean-caught fish is best; make sure the fish have fins and scales)

- All fish listed in Phase One

Poultry (pastured/organic is best)

- All poultry listed in Phase One

Eggs

- Fish roe or caviar (fresh, not preserved)

Luncheon meat (organic and nitrite/nitrate-free is best)

- Turkey, sliced (free range, preservative free)
- Roast beef, sliced (free range, preservative free)

Dairy (organic, grass-fed is best)

- Homemade kefir from raw or non-homogenized cow's milk
- Kefir from pasteurized, non-homogenized cow's milk
- Raw cow's milk hard cheeses
- Cow's milk cottage cheeses
- Cow's milk ricotta cheese
- Cow's milk plain whole-milk yogurt
- Cow's milk plain kefir
- Cow's milk plain sour cream
- Raw goat's milk

Fats and oils (organic is best)

- Expeller-pressed peanut oil

PHASE TWO

Vegetables (organic fresh or frozen is best)

* Sweet potatoes
* Yams
* Corn

Beans and legumes (soaked or fermented is best)

* White beans
* Black beans
* Kidney beans
* Navy beans
* Tempeh (fermented soybean)

Nuts and seeds (organic, raw, soaked is best)

* Walnuts (raw)
* Macadamia nuts (raw)
* Hazelnuts (raw)
* Brazil nuts (raw)
* Pecans (raw or soaked and low-temperature dehydrated)

Condiments, spices, seasonings (organic is best)

* Ketchup (no sugar)
* All-natural salad dressings (no preservatives)
* All-natural marinades (no preservatives)

Fruits (organic fresh or frozen is best)

* Apples
* Apricots
* Grapes
* Melon
* Peaches
* Oranges
* Pears
* Plums
* Kiwi

PHASE TWO

* Pineapple
* Pomegranates
* Passion fruit
* Guava

Beverages

* Raw vegetable juice (beet or carrot—maximum 50 percent of total)
* Coconut water

Sweeteners

* Unheated raw honey (up to 3 tablespoons per day)
* Stevia

Miscellaneous

* Same as Phase One

PHASE TWO: FOODS TO AVOID

Meat

* Pork
* Ham
* Bacon
* Sausage (pork)
* Ostrich
* Emu
* Imitation meat product (soy)
* Veggie burgers

Fish and seafood

* Fried, breaded fish
* Catfish
* Eel
* Squid
* Shark

* Avoid *all shellfish*, including crab, oyster, mussels, lobster, shrimp, scallops, and crawfish.

Poultry

* Fried, breaded chicken

Eggs

* Imitation eggs (such as Egg Beaters)

Luncheon meat

* Ham
* Corned beef

Dairy

* Soy milk
* Rice milk
* Almond milk
* Avoid all commercial dairy products including milk, ice cream, cheese, and yogurt.

Fats and oils

* Lard
* Margarine
* Shortening
* Soy oil
* Safflower oil
* Canola oil
* Sunflower oil
* Corn oil
* Cottonseed oil
* Any partially hydrogenated oil

Vegetables

* White potato

Beans and legumes

* Soy beans
* Tofu
* Garbanzo beans
* Lima beans

Nuts and seeds

* Peanuts
* Peanut butter
* Honey-roasted nuts
* Cashews
* Nuts or seeds roasted in oil

Condiments, spices, seasonings

* All spices that contain added sugar

Fruits

* Bananas
* Mango
* Papaya
* Canned fruit
* Avoid *dried fruits*, including raisins, dates, figs, prunes, bananas, mango, and papaya.

Beverages

* Alcoholic beverages of any kind
* Fruit juices
* Sodas
* Chlorinated tap water
* Pre-ground commercial coffee

Grains and starchy carbohydrates

* Avoid *all* grains and starchy foods in Phase Two, including bread, pasta, cereal, rice, oatmeal, pastries, and baked goods.

PHASE TWO

Sweeteners

* Sugar
* Maple syrup
* Heated honey
* Fructose and corn syrup
* All artificial sweeteners, including aspartame, sucralose, and Acesulfame K
* Sugar alcohol (including sorbitol, maltitol, and xylitol)

Miscellaneous

* Milk or whey protein powder from cow's milk
* Soy protein powder
* Rice protein powder

PHASE TWO

DAILY REGIMEN FOR PHASE TWO: DAYS 15–28

Morning hygiene

Aromatherapy A.M. (Advanced). Use three drops of a biblical aromatherapeutic blend in the palm of your hand. Rub your hands together, cup them in front of your face, and gently inhale through your nose three or four times. You may then rub the remaining oil into your scalp or into the soles of your feet.

Morning cleansing drink (intermediate)

Mix 2 tablespoons of a whole-food fiber blend and 1–2 tablespoons or 5 caplets of a green superfood blend in 8 to 12 ounces of purified water or diluted vegetable juice. Shake vigorously and drink immediately.

Morning tune-up

Recite morning prayer.

Exercise ten to fifteen minutes. Choose from functional fitness, jumping on a rebounder, performing breathing exercise, or going a walk around the neighborhood.

Listen to music that uplifts and energizes while you exercise.

Breakfast

See the sample breakfast menus in this 40-Day Plan or check out the recipes in Appendix A.

Breakfast supplements (Basic)

Whole-food multivitamin, 2–3 caplets.

Lunch

See the sample lunch menus in this 40-Day Plan or check out the recipes in Appendix A.

Lunch supplements (Basic)

Whole-food multivitamin, 2–3 caplets.

Afternoon cleansing drink (Intermediate)

Mix 2 tablespoons of a whole-food fiber blend and 1–2 tablespoons or 5 caplets of a green superfood blend in 8 to 12 ounces purified water or diluted vegetable juice. Shake vigorously and drink immediately.

Dinner

See the sample dinner menus in this 40-Day Plan or check out the recipes in Appendix A.

Dinner supplements (Basic)

Whole-food multivitamin, 2–3 caplets.

Cod liver oil (basic): 1 teaspoon to 1 tablespoon based on sun exposure. If you receive more than two hours of direct sunlight per week, you may take 1–2 teaspoons. If you receive less than two hours of direct sunlight per week, you may take 1 tablespoon.

Evening snack

See sample snack menus in this 40-Day Plan or check out the recipes in Appendix A.

Evening wind-down

Recite evening prayer.

Exercise ten to fifteen minutes. Choose from functional fitness, jumping on a rebounder, performing breathing exercise, or going on a walk around the neighborhood.

PHASE TWO

Listen to music that uplifts and energizes while you exercise.

Evening hygiene

Aromatherapy P.M. (Advanced) Use three drops of a biblical aromatherapeutic blend in the palm of your hand. Rub your hands together, cup them in front of your face, and gently inhale through your nose three or four times. You may then rub the remaining oil into your scalp or into the soles of your feet.

Healing bath (optional)

In bed before 10:30

SAMPLE MENUS FOR PHASE TWO

Day 15

Breakfast

Cottage cheese or ricotta cheese
Pineapple
Sliced almonds

Lunch

Uptown Salad

Dinner

Venison Steaks with Marinade
Sweet potatoes with butter
Steamed vegetable medley

Evening snack

Choose from an acceptable food in this 40-Day Plan.

Day 16

Breakfast

Garden Herb Omelet
1 orange

Lunch

Salade Nicoise

Dinner

Chicken with Oregano and Mushrooms
Corn on the cob

Steamed broccoli and carrots with butter

Evening snack
Apple slices

Almond butter and honey

Day 17

Breakfast
Easy Soft-boiled/Hard-boiled Eggs

Avocado with salsa

Lunch
Chicken Soup/Stock

Dinner
Red Snapper Mexican Style

Black beans

Easy Vegetable Salad

Evening snack
Mixed raw nuts (almonds, walnuts, pecans, Macadamia nuts)

Apple slices

1 ounce cheese

Day 18

Breakfast
None (partial-fast day)

Lunch
None (partial-fast day)

Dinner
Ginger Carrots

Mushroom Soup

Green salad

Grilled chicken breast

Pan-fried sweet potato in coconut oil or butter

Evening snack
None (partial-fast day)

PHASE TWO

The Maker's Diet

Phase Three: Days 29–40 (and Beyond)

THIS PHASE MARKS THE "MOUNTAINTOP EXPERIENCE," THE WINNER'S circle, the Olympic gold medal of a challenge conquered and a battle won. You will now enter Phase Three in the fifth week of the program.

Phase Three is the maintenance phase of the diet. It is specifically designed to allow and encourage healthful eating of foods from each food group. In this phase, you will reacquaint yourself with healthy grain foods and foods higher in sugars and starches, such as potatoes.

You may notice that Phase Three of the Maker's Diet does not mandate a daily snack. (I know you looked forward to them). The good news is that if you want to have a snack, you may choose one at any time—but only from the acceptable foods.

Your weight should stabilize in this phase, and you can expect other key areas of your health picture to continue to improve. Having reached this phase, you have managed to establish considerable self-control, so it should be much easier not to "cheat."

If you do venture off the Maker's Diet, perhaps during the holidays, on a vacation, or another special event such as an extravagant birthday or anniversary celebration, you can always go back to Phase One or Phase Two for a week or two to get back into the groove. This option is always available, and you will find it to be a great tool in your journey on the path that leads to health—for life!

PHASE THREE

PHASE THREE: MORE NEW FOODS TO ENJOY

Meat (grass-fed/organic is best)

- All meats listed in Phase One and Phase Two

Fish (wild freshwater/ocean-caught fish is best; make sure the fish have fins and scales)

- All fish listed in Phase One and Phase Two

Poultry (pastured/organic is best)

- All poultry listed in Phase One and Phase Two

Eggs (high omega-3/DHA or organic is best)

- All eggs listed in Phase One and Phase Two

Luncheon meat (organic is best)

- All luncheon meat listed in Phase Two

Dairy

- All dairy listed in Phase One and Phase Two

Fats and oils (organic is best)

- All fats and oils listed in Phase One and Phase Two

Vegetables (organic fresh or frozen is best)

- All vegetables listed in Phase One and Phase Two

Beans and legumes (soaked or fermented is best)

Along with beans and legumes listed in Phase One and Phase Two, add:

- Pinto beans
- Red beans
- Split peas
- Garbanzo beans
- Lima beans

* Broad beans
* Black-eyed peas
* Edamame (boiled soybeans) (in small amounts)

Nuts and seeds (organic, raw, soaked is best)
Along with nuts and seeds listed in Phase One and Phase Two, add:

* Almonds (dry roasted)
* Walnuts (dry roasted)
* Almond butter (roasted)
* Tahini (roasted)
* Pecans (dry roasted)
* Macadamia nuts (dry roasted)
* Sunflower seeds (dry roasted)
* Pumpkin seeds (dry roasted)
* Pumpkin seed butter (roasted)
* Sunflower butter (roasted)
* Peanuts, dry roasted (must be organic) (in small quantities)
* Peanut butter, roasted (must be organic) (in small quantities)
* Cashews, raw or dry roasted (in small quantities)
* Cashew butter, raw or roasted (in small quantities)

Condiments, spices, seasonings (organic is best)

* All condiments, spices, and seasonings listed in Phase One and Phase Two

Fruits (organic fresh or frozen is best)
Along with fruits listed in Phase One and Phase Two, add:

* Banana
* Mango
* Papaya
* Canned fruit (in its own juices)
* Dried fruit (no sugar or sulfites): raisins, figs, dates, prunes, pineapple, papaya, peaches, and apples

PHASE THREE

Beverages

Along with beverages listed in Phase One and Phase Two, add:

- Raw, unpasteurized vegetable juice
- Raw, unpasteurized fruit juice
- Organic wine and beer (in very small amounts)

Grains and starchy carbohydrates (whole-grain, organic, soaked is best)

- Sprouted, Ezekiel-type bread
- Sprouted Essene bread
- Fermented whole-grain sourdough bread
- Whole-grain kamut or spelt pasta (in small quantities)
- Quinoa
- Amaranth
- Buckwheat
- Millet
- Kamut (in small quantities)
- Sprouted cereal
- Oats (in small quantities)
- Spelt (in small quantities)
- Barley (in small quantities)
- Brown rice (in small quantities)

Sweeteners

Along with sweeteners listed in Phase One and Phase Two, add:

- 100 percent pure maple syrup
- Organic cane juice

Miscellaneous

- Selected healthy snacks (a few times per week)
- Trail Mix
- Organic chocolate spreads
- Carob powder
- Zesty Popcorn

Phase Three: Foods to Avoid

Meat

* Pork
* Ham
* Bacon
* Sausage (pork)
* Veggie burgers
* Ostrich
* Emu
* Imitation meat product (soy)

Fish and seafood

* Fried, breaded fish
* Catfish
* Eel
* Squid
* Shark
* Avoid *all shellfish*, including crab, oyster, mussels, lobster, shrimp, scallops, and crawfish.

Poultry

* Fried, breaded chicken

Eggs

* Imitation eggs (such as Egg Beaters)

Luncheon meat

* Ham
* Corned beef

Dairy

* Soy milk
* Rice milk
* Almond milk

* Processed cheese food or singles
* Avoid all commercial dairy products, including milk and ice cream.

Fats and oils

* Lard
* Margarine
* Shortening
* Soy oil
* Safflower oil
* Canola oil
* Sunflower oil
* Corn oil
* Cottonseed oil
* Any partially hydrogenated oil

Nuts and seeds

* Nuts roasted in oil
* Honey-roasted nuts

Condiments, spices, seasonings

* All spices that contain added sugar

Fruits

* Canned fruits in syrup

Beverages

* Fruit juices
* Sodas
* Chlorinated tap water
* Pre-ground commercial coffee
* Alcoholic beverages of any kind

Grains and starchy carbohydrates

* White rice

* Dried cereal (except sprouted)
* Instant oatmeal
* Pastries
* Baked goods
* Bread (except sprouted or sourdough)
* Pastas (except whole-grain kamut or spelt)

Sweeteners

* Sugar
* Heated honey
* Fructose or corn syrup
* Sugar alcohol, including sorbitol and xylitol
* All artificial sweeteners, including aspartame, sucralose, and Acesulfame K

Miscellaneous

* Soy protein powder
* Rice protein powder
* Milk or whey protein powder from cow's milk

DAILY REGIMEN FOR PHASE THREE: DAYS 29–40 (AND BEYOND)

Morning hygiene

Aromatherapy A.M. (Advanced). Use three drops of a biblical aromatherapeutic blend in the palm of your hand. Rub your hands together, cup them in front of your face, and gently inhale through your nose three or four times. You may then rub the remaining oil into your scalp or into the soles of your feet.

Morning cleansing drink (intermediate)

Mix 2 tablespoons of a whole-food fiber blend and 1–2 tablespoons or 5 caplets of a green superfood blend in 8 to 12 ounces of purified water or diluted vegetable juice. Shake vigorously and drink immediately.

Morning tune-up

Recite morning prayer.

PHASE THREE

Exercise fifteen to twenty minutes. Choose from functional fitness, jumping on a rebounder, performing breathing exercise, or going on a walk around the neighborhood.

Listen to music that uplifts and energizes while you exercise.

Breakfast

See the sample breakfast menus in this 40-Day Plan or check out the recipes in Appendix A.

Breakfast supplements (Basic)

Whole-food multivitamin, 2–3 caplets.

Lunch

See the sample lunch menus in this 40-Day Plan or check out the recipes in Appendix A.

Lunch supplements (Basic)

Whole-food multivitamin, 2–3 caplets.

Afternoon cleansing drink (Intermediate)

Mix 2 tablespoons of a whole-food fiber blend and 1–2 tablespoons or 5 caplets of a green superfood blend in 8 to 12 ounces purified water or diluted vegetable juice. Shake vigorously and drink immediately.

Dinner

See the sample dinner menus in this 40-Day Plan or check out the recipes in Appendix A.

Dinner supplements (Basic)

Whole-food multivitamin, 2–3 caplets.

Cod liver oil (basic): 1 teaspoon to 1 tablespoon based on sun exposure. If you receive more than two hours of direct sunlight per week, you may take 1–2 teaspoons. If you receive less than two hours of direct sunlight per week, you may take 1 tablespoon.

Evening snack

See sample snack menus in this 40-Day Plan or check out the recipes in Appendix A.

PHASE THREE

Evening wind down

Exercise fifteen to twenty minutes. Choose from functional fitness, jumping on a rebounder, performing breathing exercise, or going on a walk around the neighborhood.

Listen to music that uplifts and energizes while you exercise.

Evening hygiene

Aromatherapy P.M. (Advanced). Use three drops of a biblical aromatherapeutic blend in the palm of your hand. Rub your hands together, cup them in front of your face, and gently inhale through your nose three or four times. You may then rub the remaining oil into your scalp or into the soles of your feet.

Healing bath (optional)

In bed before 10:30

SAMPLE MENUS FOR PHASE THREE: DAYS 29-40 (AND BEYOND)

Day 29

Breakfast

Berry Smoothie

Lunch

Sliced turkey and avocado sandwich on toasted sprouted or wholegrain sourdough bread

Carrot and celery sticks

Dinner

Barbecue style chicken breast

Pan-roasted red bliss potatoes

Steamed asparagus

Day 30

Breakfast

Tomato Basil Omelet

1 orange or grapefruit

Lunch

Uptown Salad

PHASE THREE

Dinner
Lamb Chops
Baked potato with butter
Steamed vegetables (carrots, peas, broccoli)

Day 31

Breakfast
Fried eggs
Blueberry Pecan Pancakes

Lunch
Green salad
Chicken Soup/Stock

Dinner
Green salad
Easy Broiled Halibut
Steamed broccoli

Day 32

Breakfast
None (partial-fast day)

Lunch
None (partial-fast day)

Dinner
Raw Sauerkraut
Green salad
Beef Soup
Chicken Fajitas
Sprouted tortillas
Salsa, guacamole, sour cream

Evening snack
None (partial-fast day)

Appendix A

The Maker's Diet Recipes

SOUPS AND STOCKS

BEEF SOUP/STOCK

About 6 lb. beef marrow and knuckle bones	3 celery stalks, coarsely chopped
1 calf's foot, cut into pieces (optional)	Several sprigs of fresh thyme, tied together
5 lb. meaty rib or neck bones	1 tsp. dried green peppercorns, crushed
4 or more quarts cold, filtered water	1 bunch parsley
3 onions, coarsely chopped	¼ cup vinegar
3 carrots, coarsely chopped	

Good beef stock must be made with several sorts of beef bones. Knuckle bones and feet impart large quantities of gelatin to the broth; marrow bones impart flavor and the particular nutrients of the bone marrow; and meaty rib or neck bones add color and flavor.

Place the knuckle and marrow bones and calf's foot (optional) in a very large pot; cover with water. Let stand for one hour. Meanwhile, place meaty bones in a roasting pan and brown at 350 degrees in the oven. When well browned, add to the pot along with vinegar and vegetables.

Pour fat from roasting pan, add cold water, set over a high flame, and bring to a boil, stirring with a wooden spoon to de-glaze. Add this liquid to the pot. Add additional water, if necessary, to cover the bones, but the liquid should come no higher than within 1 inch of the rim of the pot, as the volume expands slightly during cooking. Bring to a boil. A large amount of scum will come to the top. It is important to remove this with a spoon. After you have skimmed, reduce heat and add the thyme and crushed peppercorns.

Simmer stock for at least 12 hours and for as long as 72 hours. Just before finishing, add the parsley. Let it wilt and remove stock from heat.

You will now have a pot of rather repulsive-looking brown liquid containing globs of gelatinous and fatty material. It doesn't even smell particularly good. But don't despair. After straining, you will have a delicious and nourishing clear broth that forms the basis for many other recipes in this book.

Remove bones with tongs or a slotted spoon. Strain the stock into a large bowl. Let cool in the refrigerator, and remove the congealed fat that rises to the top. Reheat and transfer to storage containers.

Note: Your dog will love the leftover meat and bones.

VARIATION: LAMB STOCK
Use lamb bones, especially lamb neck bones. This makes a delicious stock.

From *Nourishing Traditions* by Sally Fallon. Used by permission.

CHICKEN SOUP/STOCK

1 whole chicken (free range, pastured or organic)	6 celery stalks, coarsely chopped
2–4 chicken feet (optional)	2–4 zucchinis
3–4 quarts cold-filtered water	4–6 Tbsp. extra-virgin coconut oil
1 Tbsp. raw apple cider vinegar	1 bunch parsley
4 medium-sized onions, coarsely chopped	5 garlic cloves
8 carrots, peeled and coarsely chopped	4 inches grated ginger
	2–4 Tbsp. Celtic salt

If you are using a whole chicken, remove fat glands and gizzards from the cavity. By all means, use chicken feet if you can find them—they are full of gelatin. (Jewish folklore considers the addition of chicken feet the secret to successful broth.) Place chicken or chicken pieces in a large stainless steel pot with the water, vinegar, and all vegetables except parsley. Bring to a boil, and remove scum that rises to the top. Cover and cook on low heat for 12 to 24 hours.

The longer you cook the stock, the richer and more flavorful it will be. About five minutes before finishing the stock, add parsley. This will impart additional mineral ions to the broth.

Remove from heat, and take chicken out of pot. Let it cool, then remove meat from the carcass. Reserve for other uses such as chicken salads, enchiladas, sandwiches, or curries. (The skin and smaller bones, which will be very soft, may be given to your dog or cat.) Strain the stock into a large bowl and reserve in your refrigerator for use as a base for other soups.

VARIATIONS: TURKEY STOCK AND DUCK STOCK

Prepare as chicken stock using turkey wings and drumsticks or duck carcasses from which the breasts, legs, and thighs have been removed. These stocks will have a stronger flavor than chicken stock and will profit from the addition of several sprigs of fresh thyme tied together during cooking.

From *Nourishing Traditions* by Sally Fallon. Used by permission.

FISH STOCK

3 or 4 whole carcasses, including heads, of non-oily fish such as sole, turbot, rockfish, or snapper	Several sprigs fresh thyme
	Several sprigs parsley
2 Tbsp. extra-virgin coconut oil or butter	1 bay leaf
2 onions, coarsely chopped	½ cup dry white wine or vermouth
1 carrot, coarsely chopped	1 Tbsp. apple cider vinegar

Melt coconut oil or butter in a large stainless steel pot. Add the vegetables and cook very gently, about 30 minutes, until they are soft. Add wine and bring to a boil. Add fish carcasses and cover with cold, filtered water. Add vinegar. Bring to a boil. Take the time to carefully skim off the scum and impurities as they rise to the top. Tie herbs together and add to the pot. Reduce heat; cover and simmer for at least 4 hours or overnight. Remove carcasses with tongs or a slotted spoon, and strain the liquid into pint-sized storage containers for refrigerator or freezer.

The carrot will add a delicate sweetness to the stock when it has been reduced. Do not be tempted to add more carrots to the stock, or your final sauce will be too sweet!

From *Nourishing Traditions* by Sally Fallon. Used by permission.

COCONUT MILK SOUP

1½ quarts homemade fish or chicken stock	1 Tbsp. grated fresh ginger
1½ cups coconut milk and cream	2 Tbsp. fish sauce (optional)
1 lb. chicken or fish, cut into small cubes	2–4 Tbsp. lime juice
3 jalapeño chilies, diced, or ½ tsp. cayenne pepper, dried	Chopped cilantro for garnish

Simmer all ingredients until meat is cooked through. Garnish with cilantro. **SERVES 6–8.**

From *Nourishing Traditions* by Sally Fallon. Used by permission.

MUSHROOM SOUP

2 medium onions, peeled and chopped	1 piece toasted whole-grain sprouted or
3 Tbsp. extra-virgin coconut oil or butter	sourdough bread, broken into pieces
2 lb. fresh mushrooms	Freshly ground nutmeg
Butter and extra-virgin olive oil	Sea salt or fish sauce and pepper to taste
1 quart chicken stock	Sour cream or creme fraiche
½ cup dry white wine	

The mushrooms must be very fresh! Sauté the onions gently in extra-virgin coconut oil or butter until soft. Meanwhile, wash mushrooms (no need to remove stems) and dry well. Cut into quarters. In a heavy cast-iron skillet, sauté the mushrooms in small batches in a mixture of butter and olive oil. Remove with slotted spoon and drain on paper towels. Add sautéed mushrooms, wine, bread, and chicken stock to onions; bring to a boil, and then skim. Reduce heat and simmer about 15 minutes.

Blend soup with a handheld blender. Add nutmeg and season to taste. Ladle into heated soup bowls and serve with cultured cream. **SERVES 6.**

From *Nourishing Traditions* by Sally Fallon. Used by permission.

RED MEAT CHILI

3 lb. coarsely ground beef, buffalo, or game	1 Tbsp. ground cumin
Extra-virgin olive oil	2 Tbsp. dried oregano
¼ cup red wine	2 Tbsp. dried basil
2 cups homemade beef stock	¼ to ½ tsp. red chili flakes
2 onions, finely chopped	4 cups cooked, soaked kidney beans
2–4 small green chilies, hot or mild, seeded	No-oil chips for garnish
and chopped	Chopped green onions for garnish
2 cans tomatoes, briefly chopped in food	Creme fraiche or sour cream for garnish
processor	Avocado slices for garnish
3 cloves garlic, peeled and mashed	Chopped cilantro for garnish

Brown meat until crumbly in a little olive oil in a heavy pot. (Olive oil may not be necessary if the beef contains a lot of fat.) Add remaining ingredients. Simmer about 1 hour. Serve with garnishes. **SERVES 8–12.**

From *Nourishing Traditions* by Sally Fallon. Used by permission.

SALADS

EASY VEGETABLE SALAD

1 head romaine, Boston, or red lettuce (or mixed greens)	2 plum tomatoes, seeded and chopped
½ zucchini, quartered	½ red onion, sliced
½ cucumber, quartered	2–3 oz. raw cheddar cheese, grated
	Dressing of your choice

Place enough lettuce to cover the bottom of your salad bowl, then add a layer each of the other items, then another layer of lettuce, repeating until all ingredients are used up. Serve the dressing on the side, or mix into the entire salad and serve. **SERVES 4.**

From *The Lazy Person's Whole Food Cookbook* by Stephen Byrnes. Used by permission.

UPTOWN SALAD

Romaine, Boston, red lettuce, or mixed greens	½ red onion, sliced
4 oz. turkey breast or roast beef	½ avocado, sliced
½ red pepper	2–3 oz. Gorgonzola cheese, grated
½ cucumber, quartered	Dressing of your choice
1 tomato, sliced	

SERVES 1.

By Brian Upton. Used by permission.

ITALIAN SALAD

1 head romaine	1 small red onion, finely sliced
1 bunch watercress	½ cup small seed sprouts
1 red pepper, seeded and cut into a julienne	2 carrots, peeled and grated
1 cucumber, peeled, seeded, quartered lengthwise, and finely sliced	1 cup red cabbage, finely shredded
1 heart of celery with leaves, finely chopped	1 cup cooked chickpeas
	¾ cup Basic Salad Dressing (page 237) or garlic dressing

This is a good, basic salad. Children love it. The secret is to cut everything up small. Remove the outer leaves of the romaine, slice off the end, and open up to rinse out any dirt or impurities, while keeping the head intact. Pat dry. Slice across at ½-inch intervals. Place romaine in your salad bowl, then watercress, then add chopped vegetables in different piles. Finally strew sprouts and garbanzo beans over the top for an attractive presentation. Bring to the table to show off your creation before tossing with dressing. May be served with grated Parmesan cheese. **SERVES 6.**

VARIATION: MEXICAN SALAD

Use Mexican dressing rather than Basic Salad Dressing or garlic dressing. Omit chickpeas. Top with a sprinkle of pepitas, or thin strips of sprouted wheat tortillas, sautéed in olive oil until crisp.

From *Nourishing Traditions* by Sally Fallon. Used by permission.

ORIENTAL RED MEAT SALAD

1½ lb. beef flank steak, or similar cut from lamb or game	1 tsp. grated fresh ginger
½ cup lemon juice	Pinch of red pepper flakes
6 Tbsp. soy sauce	2 Tbsp. toasted sesame seeds
2 Tbsp. extra-virgin olive oil or expeller-expressed peanut oil	½ lb. snow peas, steamed lightly and cut into quarters at an angle
1 Tbsp. toasted sesame oil	1 pound bean sprouts, steamed lightly
	1 red pepper, seeded and cut into a julienne

Using a sharp knife, score the flank steak or red meat pieces across the grain on both sides. Broil 3 or 4 minutes to a side, or until meat is medium rare. Transfer to a cutting board and let stand for 10 minutes. Meanwhile, mix lemon juice, soy sauce, oils, ginger, and red pepper flakes together. Cut the meat across the grain on an angle into very thin slices, then cut these slices into a julienne. Marinate with soy sauce mixture for several hours in refrigerator. Mix with sesame seeds and vegetables just before serving. **SERVES 6.**

From *Nourishing Traditions* by Sally Fallon. Used by permission.

SALADE NICOISE

6 portions fresh tuna steak, about 4 ounces each Extra-virgin olive oil 6 cups baby salad greens or frise lettuce 6 small ripe tomatoes, cut into wedges 6 small red potatoes, cooked in a clay pot	1 lb. French beans, blanched for 8 minutes and rinsed under cold water 2 dozen small black olives 2 cups herb dressing, made with finely chopped parsley

Brush tuna steaks with olive oil, and season with sea salt and pepper. Using a heavy skillet, cook rapidly, two at a time, for about 4 minutes per side. Set aside.

Divide salad greens between 6 large plates. Garnish with tomatoes, potatoes, beans, and olives. Place steaks on top of greens. Add dressing. This is delicious with sourdough bread or pizza toasts. **SERVES 6.**

From *Nourishing Traditions* by Sally Fallon. Used by permission.

TUNA TAHINI SALAD

2 large cans water-packed tuna, drained and flaked ¼ tsp. cayenne pepper 2 cups tahini sauce (see below) 4 medium onions, thinly sliced	Melted butter and extra-virgin olive oil 1/3 cup toasted pine nuts Cilantro sprigs for garnish Toasted, sprouted, or sourdough bread or sprouted crackers

Mix tuna with cayenne pepper and 1 cup sauce. Meanwhile, strew the onions on an oiled cookie sheet; brush with mixture of melted butter and olive oil, and bake at 375 degrees until crisp. Mound tuna on a platter. Scatter onions and pine nuts on top. Garnish with cilantro, and serve with dehydrated, sprouted, whole-grain crackers and remaining sauce. **SERVES 6–8.**

From *Nourishing Traditions* by Sally Fallon. Used by permission.

TAHINI SAUCE

2 cloves garlic, peeled and coarsely chopped 1 tsp. sea salt ½ cup tahini	1 Tbsp. unrefined flaxseed oil 1 cup water ½ cup fresh lemon juice

Place garlic in food processor with salt. Blend until minced. Add tahini and flaxseed oil and blend. Using attachment that allows addition of liquids drop by drop and with motor running, add water. When completely blended, add lemon juice all at once and blend until smooth. Sauce should be the consistency of heavy cream. If too thick, add more water and lemon juice. **MAKES 2 CUPS.**

From *Nourishing Traditions* by Sally Fallon. Used by permission.

VEGETABLES

General preparation guidelines: Do not boil vegetables unless this is required to eat them. Steam your veggies for a few minutes, then add butter or ghee, seasonings, and serve. You can also sauté your vegetables in extra-virgin coconut oil. Raw veggies with a healthy dressing or dip are also good.

EASY SAUTÉED GREENS

1 quart spinach or other greens Extra-virgin coconut oil	Sea salt/pepper to taste

Wash the spinach or greens in several waters. Remove all stems and brown leaves. Heat extra-virgin coconut oil in skillet. Place leaves in the skillet and cover. Cook till wilted, stirring occasionally. Season as you like. **SERVES 6–8.**

From *The Lazy Person's Whole Food Cookbook* by Stephen Byrnes. Used by permission.

CULTURED VEGETABLES

GINGER CARROTS

4 cups grated carrots, loosely packed 1 Tbsp. fresh ginger, grated 2 tsp. sea salt	2 Tbsp. whey (if not available, add an additional 1 tsp. salt)

This is the best introduction to lacto-fermented vegetables we know. The taste is delicious, and the sweetness of the carrots neutralizes the acidity that some people find disagreeable when first introduced to lacto-fermented vegetables. Ginger carrots go well with fish and with highly spiced meats.

In a bowl, mix all ingredients and pound with wooden pounder to release juices. Place in a quart-sized, wide-mouth Mason jar and press down with the wooden pounder. There should be about an inch of space between the top of carrots and the top of the jar. Cover tightly. Leave at room temperature about 2–3 days before transferring to cold storage. **MAKES 1 QUART.**

From *Nourishing Traditions* by Sally Fallon. Used by permission.

RAW SAUERKRAUT

4 cups shredded cabbage, loosely packed ½ tsp. cumin seeds ½ tsp. mustard seeds	2 tsp. Celtic sea salt 2 Tbsp. homemade whey 1 cup filtered water

In a bowl, mix cabbage with cumin and mustard seeds. Mash or pound with a wooden pounder for several minutes to release juices. Place in a quart-sized, wide-mouthed Mason jar and pack down with the pounder. Mix water with sea salt and whey, and pour into jar. Add more water if needed to bring liquid to top of cabbage. There should be about one inch of space between the top of cabbage and the top of the jar. Cover tightly, and keep at room temperature for about 3 days. Transfer to cold storage. The sauerkraut can be eaten immediately, but it improves with age. **MAKES 1 QUART.**

From *Nourishing Traditions* by Sally Fallon. Used by permission.

SAUCES, DRESSINGS, DIPS

BASIC SALAD DRESSING

½ cup extra-virgin olive oil	1 tsp. Dijon-type mustard
1 Tbsp. unrefined flaxseed oil	Herbamare seasoning to taste
2 Tbsp. apple cider vinegar or lemon juice	

Combine all ingredients and blend slowly. **MAKES ABOUT ¾ CUP.**

Adapted from *Nourishing Traditions* by Sally Fallon. Used by permission.

BALSAMIC DRESSING

1 tsp. Dijon-type dressing, smooth or grainy	½ cup extra-virgin olive oil
2 Tbsp. plus 1 tsp. balsamic vinegar	1 Tbsp. unrefined flaxseed oil

Balsamic vinegar is a red wine vinegar that has been aged in wooden casks. It has a delicious, pungent flavor that goes well with dark greens such as watercress or mache. Prepare as in Basic Salad Dressing recipe. **MAKES ABOUT ¾ CUP.**

From *Nourishing Traditions* by Sally Fallon. Used by permission.

BARBECUE SAUCE

¾ cup teriyaki sauce	¾ cup naturally sweetened ketchup

Mix ketchup into teriyaki sauce with a whisk. **MAKES 1½ CUPS.**

From *Nourishing Traditions* by Sally Fallon. Used by permission.

BETTER BUTTER

½ cup raw or organic butter (unsalted)	½ cup flaxseed or hempseed oil
½ cup extra-virgin coconut oil	¼ tsp. fine Celtic sea salt

Allow butter and coconut oil to soften at room temperature. Combine with flaxseed or hempseed oil, and add salt. Refrigerate and use as a spread. Note: Never use Better Butter for cooking. The essential fatty acids contained in the oil will be damaged by the heat. **MAKES 1½ CUPS.**

By Jordan Rubin

CREAMY AVOCADO DIP

1 ripe avocado, peeled and cut into pieces	Juice of 1 lemon
3 anchovy fillets (optional)	2 tsp. unrefined flaxseed oil
½ cup sour cream or creme fraiche	1 clove garlic, mashed

Place all ingredients in food processor and blend until smooth. Chill well before serving. Serve with vegetable sticks or baked tortillas, broken into chips. **MAKES 1½ CUPS.**

From *Nourishing Traditions* by Sally Fallon. Used by permission.

CREAMY DRESSING

¾ cup Basic Salad Dressing (page237)	¼ cup sour cream, yogurt, or kefir

This is a traditional recipe of the Auvergne region of France. Prepare Basic Salad Dressing. Blend in cream with a fork. **MAKES ABOUT 1 CUP.**

From *Nourishing Traditions* by Sally Fallon. Used by permission.

EASY AVOCADO DRESSING

1 ripe avocado	2 Tbsp. extra-virgin olive oil
1 stalk of celery	Herbamare seasoning to taste
1 small red pepper, seeded	

Blend avocado together with oil, celery, and pepper slices in blender until smooth.

From *The Lazy Person's Whole Food Cookbook* by Stephen Byrnes. Used by permission.

EASY FRENCH DRESSING

½ cup high-oleic safflower, sunflower, or walnut oil	¼ tsp. Herbamare seasoning
	¼ tsp. paprika
4 Tbsp. raw apple cider vinegar or lemon juice	Few grains of cayenne pepper
2 tsp. raw, unheated honey	

Combine dry ingredients and apple cider vinegar or lemon juice. Add oil slowly, beating constantly until thick.

From *The Lazy Person's Whole Food Cookbook* by Stephen Byrnes. Used by permission.

GUACAMOLE

2 ripe avocados	2 Tbsp. cilantro, finely chopped (optional)
Juice of 1 lemon	Pinch Celtic sea salt or Herbamare

Peel avocados. Place flesh in a bowl and squeeze lemon juice over it. Use a fork to mash (do not use a food processor). Guacamole should be slightly lumpy. Stir in the cilantro. Guacamole should be made just before serving as it will turn dark in an hour or two. Serve with vegetable sticks or baked tortillas, broken into chips. **MAKES 1½ CUPS.**

From *Nourishing Traditions* by Sally Fallon. Used by permission.

HERB DRESSING

¾ cup Basic Salad Dressing (page 237)	1 tsp. very finely chopped fresh herbs such as parsley, tarragon, thyme, basil, or oregano

Prepare Basic Salad Dressing and stir in herbs. **MAKES ABOUT ¾ CUP.**

From *Nourishing Traditions* by Sally Fallon. Used by permission.

ORIENTAL DRESSING

2 Tbsp. rice vinegar	1 clove garlic, peeled and mashed (optional)
1 Tbsp. soy sauce	½ tsp. raw honey
1 tsp. grated ginger	½ cup extra-virgin olive oil
1 tsp. toasted sesame oil	1 tsp. unrefined flaxseed oil
1 tsp. finely chopped green onion or chives	

Place all ingredients in a jar and shake vigorously. **MAKES ABOUT ½ CUP.**

From *Nourishing Traditions* by Sally Fallon. Used by permission.

SALSA

4 medium tomatoes, peeled, seeded, and diced	Juice of 2 lemons
2 small onions, finely diced	2 tsp. Celtic sea salt
¼ cup diced chili pepper, hot or mild	2 Tbsp. whey (if not available, use an additional
1 bunch cilantro, chopped	1 tsp. salt)
1 tsp. dried oregano	½–1 cup filtered water

Mix all ingredients except water, and place in a quart-sized, wide-mouth Mason jar. Press down lightly with a wooden pounder. Add enough water to cover vegetables. Cover tightly and keep at room temperature for 2 days before transferring to cold storage. **MAKES 1 QUART.**

From *Nourishing Traditions* by Sally Fallon. Used by permission.

TERIYAKI SAUCE

1 Tbsp. grated fresh ginger	1 Tbsp. rice vinegar
3 garlic cloves, mashed	1 Tbsp. raw honey
1 Tbsp. toasted sesame oil	½ cup soy sauce

Use as a marinade for chicken or duck. Mix all ingredients together with a whisk. **MAKES ¾ CUP.**

From *Nourishing Traditions* by Sally Fallon. Used by permission.

YOGURT TAHINI INBETWEENI

4 oz. Probiogurt	Juice of one freshly squeezed lemon
1 Tbsp. Dijon-style mustard	1 Tbsp. raw tahini (sesame butter)
1 Tbsp. yellow or brown mustard	½ tsp. of fine Celtic sea salt

Combine all ingredients together and mix thoroughly.

By Jason Dewberry. Used by permission.

EGGS

EASY SCRAMBLED EGGS

6 eggs	3 Tbsp. melted butter or extra virgin coconut oil
Celtic sea salt, pepper	Few grains of cayenne pepper (optional)
¼ cup heavy cream	

Beat eggs well. Add cream. Heat butter in skillet or pan; add egg mixture, cooking slowly, until of a creamy texture. If desired, 1 cup of chopped turkey bacon, chicken, beef, or peppers may be added for variations in taste. **SERVES 3–4.**

From *The Lazy Person's Whole Food Cookbook* by Stephen Byrnes. Used by permission.

EASY SOFT-BOILED/HARDBOILED EGGS

Wash eggs and cover with boiling water. Simmer for 4 minutes if you're making soft-boiled eggs, and 12 minutes if you're making hardboiled eggs. Hardboiled eggs may be plunged into cold water if you will be using them in another recipe, such as sliced additions or garnishes. Hardboiled eggs may also be made several at a time and then refrigerated for convenient snacking later.

From *The Lazy Person's Whole Food Cookbook* by Stephen Byrnes. Used by permission.

BASIC OMELET

4 fresh eggs, at room temperature	Pinch sea salt
3 Tbsp. extra-virgin coconut oil or butter	

Crack eggs into a bowl. Add water and sea salt, and blend with a wire whisk. (Do not over-whisk or the omelet will be tough). Melt coconut oil or butter in a well-seasoned cast iron skillet or frying pan. When foam subsides, add egg mixture. Tip pan to allow egg to cover the entire pan. Cook several minutes over medium heat until underside is lightly browned. Lift up one side with a spatula and fold omelet in half. Reduce heat and cook another 30 seconds or so—this will allow the egg on the inside to cook. Slide omelet onto a heated platter and serve. **SERVES 2.**

VARIATION: ONION, PEPPER, AND GOAT CHEESE OMELET
Sauté 1 small onion, thinly sliced, and ½ red pepper, cut into julienne strips, in a little extra-virgin coconut oil or butter until tender. Strew this evenly over the egg mixture as it begins to cook, along with 2 ounces of goat's milk cheddar or feta cheese.

VARIATION: GARDEN HERB OMELET
Scatter 1 tablespoon parsley, finely chopped, 1 tablespoon chives, finely chopped, and 1 tablespoon thyme or other garden herb, finely chopped, over omelet as it begins to cook.

VARIATION: MUSHROOM SWISS OMELET
Sauté ½ pound fresh mushrooms, washed, well dried, and thinly sliced, in extra-virgin coconut oil or butter and olive oil. Scatter mushrooms and grated Swiss cheese over the omelet as it begins to cook.

VARIATION: SAUSAGE AND PEPPER OMELET
Sauté ¼ cup turkey or buffalo sausage and red or yellow peppers in a little extra-virgin coconut oil or butter until crumbly. Scatter over the omelet as it begins to cook.

VARIATION: SPINACH AND FETA OMELET
Add chopped onion to beaten eggs. Add more onions, spinach, tomatoes, and feta cheese as it begins to cook.

VARIATION: TOMATO BASIL OMELET
Scatter ¼ cup diced tomato and chopped fresh basil over omelet as it begins to cook.

From *Nourishing Traditions* by Sally Fallon. Used by permission.

VEGETABLE FRITTATA

1 cup broccoli flowerets, steamed until tender and broken into small pieces	1/3 cup sour cream or creme fraiche
1 red pepper; seeded and cut into a julienne	1 tsp. finely grated lemon rind
1 medium onion, peeled and finely chopped	Pinch dried oregano
Butter and extra-virgin olive oil	Pinch dried rosemary
6 eggs	Sea salt and freshly ground pepper
	1 cup grated raw Monterey jack cheese

In a cast iron skillet, sauté the pepper and onion in butter and olive oil until soft. Remove with a slotted spoon. Beat eggs with cream and seasonings. Stir in broccoli, peppers, and onion. Melt more butter and olive oil in the pan and pour in egg mixture. Cook over medium heat about 5 minutes until underside is golden. Sprinkle cheese on top and place under the broiler for a few minutes until the frittata puffs and browns. Cut into wedges and serve. **SERVES 4.**

From *Nourishing Traditions* by Sally Fallon. Used by permission. For variations of this recipe, order a copy of *Nourishing Traditions*. (See Appendix B.)

FISH

SIMPLE BAKED FISH

1½ lb. filet of white fish such as sole, whiting, or turbot Juice of 1 lemon	1 Tbsp. fish sauce (optional) Dash cayenne pepper 1 Tbsp. snipped fresh herbs

Place fish in buttered baking dish. Sprinkle with lemon juice, cayenne, fish sauce, herbs, and salt. Cover baking dish with foil (but don't let foil touch the fish). Bake at 300 degrees for about 15 minutes. **SERVES 4.**

From *Nourishing Traditions* by Sally Fallon. Used by permission.

EASY BROILED HALIBUT

1–2 lb. halibut Lemon juice Butter or extra-virgin coconut oil	Sea salt or Herbamare Pepper

Wipe halibut slices with damp cloth and sprinkle with salt, pepper, and lemon juice. Dot with oil or butter. Broil under high heat, turning frequently till brown. **SERVES 6–8.**

From *The Lazy Person's Whole Food Cookbook* by Stephen Byrnes. Used by permission.

EASY SMOTHERED SALMON

2 cups canned salmon ¾ cup diced celery 2 slices turkey bacon, chopped ½ cup boiling water	2 Tbsp. melted extra-virgin coconut oil or butter ¾ cup onion, chopped 1 tsp. sea salt 2 thin slices lemon (optional)

Combine oil or butter, turkey bacon, celery, onion, and salt; fry until light brown. Place salmon in center of greased baking pan. Arrange vegetables and turkey bacon around salmon. Add water and cover. Bake at 375 degrees for 30 minutes. Remove cover and cook another 10 minutes. **SERVES 6.**

From T*he Lazy Person's Whole Food Cookbook* by Stephen Byrnes. Used by permission. For more salmon recipes, order a copy of this cookbook.

SALMON SALAD

1 can water-packed salmon 1 Tbsp. omega-3 mayonnaise 1 Tbsp. flaxseed oil or garlic-chili flax	Chopped onions Chopped peppers Chopped celery

Combine all ingredients and serve over lettuce or toasted sprouted bread. **SERVES 1–2.**

By Jordan Rubin

WILD ALASKAN SALMON WITH PECAN PESTO

4 wild Alaskan salmon fillets (about 1.25–1.5 lb.) 1/3 lb. shelled pecans 3 oz. butter, cold 2–3 fresh jalapeños 1 small lemon or orange	1 3-inch sprig of rosemary Olive oil Celtic sea salt Pepper

Heat oven to 300 degrees and toast pecans on a cookie sheet until you can smell the aroma of toasted pecans, about 20-30 minutes. Transfer to a cool cookie sheet. Rinse salmon and pat dry. Butterfly fillets with a sharp knife if desired. Rub salmon with olive oil; salt and pepper both sides. Heat iron skillet or other heavy skillet over medium heat. Sauté fillets until firm to the touch.

Prepare jalapeños by removing the tops and splitting lengthwise. De-rib and remove the seeds with a sharp knife. Chop coarsely. Cut the cold butter into 1/2 Tbsp. pats. Prepare the zest of 1/2 small lemon (or orange) and chop finely. Chop the rosemary into very fine pieces. Add the butter, chopped jalapeños, pecans, rosemary, and lemon zest to a food processor. Process for 5–8 seconds and scrape the bowl. Repeat 2–3 times until a paste has formed. Do not over-process. Spread the pesto over the cooked salmon. **SERVES 4.**

By Keith Tindall from White Egret Farm. Used by permission.

FILLET OF SOLE WITH GREEN GRAPES

1 lb. sole or flounder fillets	¾ cup white wine
Celtic sea salt	¼ lb. seedless green grapes
1 Tbsp. lime juice	1 ½ Tbsp. butter
1 tsp. parsley, finely minced	1 Tbsp. whole-grain flour (soaked)
½ tsp. tarragon, finely minced	2 Tbsp. orange juice
½ clove garlic, minced	

Rinse the fillets and pat dry. Sprinkle fillets with salt and lime juice. Place in a lightly greased skillet. Sprinkle the fillets with the parsley, tarragon, and garlic. Add the wine and simmer for 12 to 15 minutes until the fish flake easily and look milky white but not transparent. Add the grapes the last 5 minutes. Remove fish from the heat and keep warm on a platter. In the original skillet, melt the butter with the remaining juices. Blend in the flour until smooth. Add the orange juice and cook, stirring until the mixture thickens. Add more wine to adjust the consistency. Pour this sauce over the fillets. **SERVES 3–4.**

By Keith Tindall from White Egret Farm. Used by permission.

RED SNAPPER MEXICAN STYLE

4 red snapper fillets	1 bunch cilantro, chopped
2 Tbsp. lime juice	1 tsp. fresh chili pepper, diced
Extra-virgin olive oil	2 cloves garlic, peeled and mashed
1 medium onion, thinly sliced	Pinch of cinnamon
2 ripe tomatoes, peeled, seeded, and chopped	Sea salt

Rub fillets with lime juice; let stand, covered, in refrigerator for several hours.

Using a heavy skillet, sauté the fillets in a little olive oil briefly, on both sides. Transfer to an oiled Pyrex baking dish. Add more olive oil to the skillet. Sauté onion until soft. Add remaining ingredients and simmer for about 30 minutes or more until most of liquid is absorbed. Season to taste with sea salt. Strew the sauce over fish and bake at 350 degrees until tender, about 25 minutes. **SERVES 4.**

From *Nourishing Traditions* by Sally Fallon. Used by permission.

TUNA STEAKS, ORIENTAL STYLE

2 lb. tuna steak, about 1 inch thick	1 Tbsp. raw, unheated honey
Extra-virgin olive oil	½ cup rice vinegar
Sea salt and freshly ground pepper	2 Tbsp. fish sauce (optional)
3 cloves garlic, peeled	1 Tbsp. toasted sesame oil
¼ cup fresh ginger, peeled and coarsely chopped	⅓ cup extra-virgin coconut oil
2 Tbsp. Dijon-type mustard	1 bunch green onions, chopped
¼ cup soy sauce	3 Tbsp. sesame seeds, toasted in oven

Brush tuna steaks with coconut oil and sprinkle with salt and pepper. Grill about 5 minutes per side on a barbecue or under a broiler. Transfer to a heated platter and keep warm until ready to serve. Meanwhile, place garlic, ginger, mustard, fish sauce, and soy sauce in food processor; process until blended. Add honey and vinegar and process again. With motor running, add oil gradually so that sauce emulsifies and becomes thick.

Place tuna steak servings on warmed plates. Spoon sauce over and garnish with green onions and sesame seeds. This dish goes well with spinach, chard, Chinese peas, or steamed Chinese cabbage. **SERVES 6.**

From *Nourishing Traditions* by Sally Fallon. Used by permission. For more tuna recipes, order a copy of *Nourishing Traditions*. (See Appendix B.)

TUNA SALAD

1 can water-packed tuna	Chopped onions
1 Tbsp. omega-3 mayonnaise	Chopped peppers
1 Tbsp. flaxseed oil or garlic-chili flax	Chopped celery

Combine all ingredients and serve over lettuce or on toasted sprouted bread. **SERVES 1–2.**

By Jordan Rubin

FOWL

CHICKEN SALAD

6 oz. chopped chicken	Chopped onions
1 Tbsp. omega-3 mayonnaise	Chopped peppers
1 Tbsp. flaxseed oil or garlic-chili flax	Chopped celery

Combine all ingredients and serve over lettuce or on toasted sprouted bread. **SERVES 1–2.**

By Jordan Rubin

CHICKEN WITH OREGANO AND MUSHROOMS

1 broiler, cut in pieces (pasture fed)	1 clove garlic, minced
¼ cup olive oil	2 tomatoes, peeled and quartered
½ cup onion, chopped	½ cup dry white wine
1 tsp. salt	8 oz. fresh mushrooms, sliced
⅛ tsp. pepper	¼ cup parsley, chopped for garnish
¼ tsp. oregano, dried, or ½ tsp. fresh oregano, finely chopped	

Brown the chicken pieces slowly in hot olive oil. Add onion, and cook until soft. Drain the oil, and season chicken with salt and pepper. Add oregano, garlic, wine, and mushrooms. Scrape the bottom of the pan to loosen browned bits. Cover and cook over low heat until the chicken is tender, about 35 minutes. Add tomatoes. Continue cooking for 5 more minutes. Garnish with parsley. **SERVES 4.**

By Keith Tindall from White Egret Farm. Used by permission.

CILANTRO LIME CHICKEN CACCIATORE

2 lb. chicken breast sliced into 1-oz. cubes	2 Tbsp. extra-virgin olive oil
1 Tbsp. minced garlic	5 medium-sized Roma tomatoes
½ cup freshly squeezed lime juice	Celtic sea salt to taste
3 Tbsp. chopped cilantro	Cayenne pepper to taste

Heat sauté pan to medium. Add olive oil, garlic, cilantro, and ¼ cup of lime juice. Simmer for 4–6 minutes. While simmering, pour ¼ cup of lime juice over chicken; let stand for 1–2 minutes. Season chicken with salt and cayenne pepper. After 4–6 minutes, add seasoned chicken to the pan and cook for 8–10 minutes over medium to medium-high heat. **SERVES 4.**

By Jason Dewberry. Used by permission.

EASY CURRIED CHICKEN

2 cups diced cooked chicken	1 Tbsp. curry powder
2 cups coconut milk/cream	1 tsp. chopped onion
4 Tbsp. butter	½ cup lemon juice
3 Tbsp. whole-grain flour (soaked)	Sea salt and pepper to taste

Melt butter, then add flour and curry powder; cook for 5 minutes. Pour in coconut milk/cream and stir well until boiling. Add the onion, then put in the chicken seasonings and heat. Add lemon juice when ready to serve. Goes great with brown rice and vegetables. **SERVES 6.**

From *The Lazy Person's Whole Food Cookbook* by Stephen Byrnes. Used by permission. For more chicken recipes, order a copy of this cookbook (www.powerhealth.net).

CHICKEN FAJITAS

2 lb. chicken breast cut into strips, about ¼ to ½ inch thick	1 green pepper, seeded and cut into julienne strips
6 Tbsp. extra-virgin olive oil	2 medium onions, thinly sliced
½ cup lemon or lime juice	Extra-virgin olive oil
¼ cup pineapple juice (optional)	12 sprouted whole-wheat tortillas
4 garlic cloves, peeled and mashed	Melted butter
½ tsp. chili powder	Crème fraiche or sour cream for garnish
1 tsp. dried oregano	Chismole for garnish
½ tsp. dried thyme	Guacamole for garnish
1 red pepper, seeded and cut into julienne strips	

Make a mixture of oil, lemon or lime juice, pineapple juice, and spices; mix well with the meat. Marinate for several hours. Remove with a slotted spoon to paper towels and pat dry. Using a heavy skillet, sauté the meat, a batch at a time, in olive oil, transferring to a heated platter and keeping warm in the oven. Meanwhile, mix vegetables in marinade. Sauté vegetables in batches in olive oil and strew over meat. Heat tortillas briefly in a heavy cast-iron skillet and brush with melted butter. Serve meat mixture with tortillas and garnishes. **SERVES 4–6.**

From *Nourishing Traditions* by Sally Fallon. Used by permission. For more chicken recipes, order a copy of this cookbook (www.powerhealth.net).

SPICY CHICKEN STUFFED PEPPERS

2 free-range chicken breasts	½ cup sharp cheddar cheese, shredded
2 Tbsp. stick of butter	2–4 red or yellow bell peppers (either whole or halves)
1 cup organic brown rice	1 slice sprouted or sourdough whole-grain bread
½ cup diced jalapeños (optional)	
2 cups or cans organic black beans	
2 Tbsp. soy sauce	

Bake chicken breasts at 450 degrees for 30 minutes. After 15 minutes of cooking, baste with butter. Bring 2½ cups of water and 1 cup of brown rice to a boil (if brown rice was soaked overnight, add additional water to make approximately 2½ cups). Stir once, and then let simmer for 45 minutes. Add diced jalapeño peppers and shredded cheese to black beans; and cook on low heat. Add soy sauce to bean mixture, stirring occasionally. Take chicken out of oven and slice. Add to the bean mixture and simmer for 15 minutes. Mix brown rice into bean mixture and chicken and mix well. Cut the tops off of the peppers or cut in halves; place desired amount of stuffing into them. Slice the bread and place on top of stuffed peppers. Bake in oven at 450 degrees for 15 minutes. Serve warm. **SERVES 2–4.** By Sherry Dewberry. Used by permission.

ROASTED PASTURED CHICKEN

1 pastured chicken, whole, 4–5 lb. (a broiler)	1 3-inch sprig rosemary
1 apple, small	Olive oil
1 onion, small	Celtic sea salt
1 stalk celery, plus leaves	Pepper, freshly ground

Rinse and drain the chicken. If you are starting with a frozen chicken, be certain it is completely thawed. Preheat the oven to 350 degrees. Quarter and core the apple. Peel and quarter onion. Slice celery into 2- to 3-inch pieces. Add about 2 Tbsp. olive oil to the cavity of the bird. Stuff bird with apple, celery, onion, and rosemary. Rub the outside of the bird with olive oil. Sprinkle bird with salt and freshly ground pepper, and rub them into the skin. Place chicken in a baking dish with 2" sides. Bake approximately 1½ hours or until a meat thermometer reads 180 degrees when pushed into the thigh. Remove the chicken from the oven and allow to rest for approximately 20 minutes before carving. The rest period allows the juices to redistribute and results in more tender meat. **SERVES 4.** By Keith Tindall from White Egret Farm. Used by permission.

WILD DUCK

4–6 ducks, preferably wild, or 2 domestic ducks may be used	4–6 sprigs of celery leaves
1 small onion	4–6 pats of extra-virgin coconut butter
1 apple, small to medium in size	1–2 cups dry wine, such as a Chardonnay

Preheat the oven to 325 degrees. Rinse and drain the ducks. Quarter the apple and onion and cut each quarter into thirds. Place one pat of butter into the cavity of each duck. Add a sprig of celery leaves, and then one or two of the apple and onion slices to fill the cavity. Place the stuffed duck breast down on a large piece of foil (the size of a cookie sheet for a small wild duck). Fold the foil to make a tight packet, leaving one end open. Add¼ to ½ cup wine to the packet, depending on the size of the duck. Close the packet. Place each packet in the Dutch oven (breast down). Cover with the lid and place into the preheated oven. The ducks should bake for 2–3 hours depending on size. DO NOT open the lid or the packets until done. The ducks are done when they feel soft. The ducks must steam inside the packets in an airtight pan to become tender. Opening the lid or the packets will allow the steam to escape. For ideal results, ducks must bake long and slow under relatively low heat. **SERVES 4.**

By Keith Tindall from White Egret Farm. Used by permission.

RED MEAT AND GAME

ALL-DAY BEEF STEW

3 lb. beef stew, cut into 1-inch pieces	Several sprigs fresh thyme, tied together
1 cup red wine	2 cloves garlic, peeled and crushed
3–4 cups beef stock	2–3 small pieces orange peel
4 tomatoes, peeled, seeded, and chopped (or 1 can tomatoes)	8 small red potatoes
2 Tbsp. tomato puree	1 pound carrots, peeled and cut into sticks
½ tsp. black peppercorns	Celtic sea salt and freshly ground pepper

This recipe is ideal for working mothers. The ingredients can be assembled in about 15 minutes in the morning—or even the night before. Marinate meat in red wine overnight. (This step is optional.) Place all ingredients except potatoes and carrots in an oven-proof casserole and cook at 250 degrees for 12 hours. Add carrots and potatoes during the last hour. Season to taste. **SERVES 6–8.**
From *Nourishing Traditions* by Sally Fallon. Used by permission.

CHEVON MEAT LOAF

1 lb. ground chevon (goat, preferably grass fed)	2 eggs
1 lb. ground beef (preferably grass fed)	1 tsp. ground thyme
½ onion, finely chopped	¼ tsp. Celtic sea salt
1 small green pepper, finely chopped	⅛ tsp. black pepper
⅔ cup bread crumbs (from sprouted or sour dough whole-grain bread)	1 cup tomato ketchup

Preheat oven to 325 degrees. Add all the ingredients to a large bowl. Mix with your hands until all the ingredients are thoroughly combined. The mixture should feel slightly sticky. Add the mixture to a baking pan with 2-inch sides, and form it into a loaf. Make an indentation longitudinally along the top of the loaf. Fill this with additional tomato ketchup. Bake at 325 degrees for approximately 1¼ hours until the loaf appears slightly brown on top. Test for doneness by checking for an internal temperature of 160 degrees. Allow the loaf to rest before slicing in order to avoid crumbling. **SERVES 4–6.**
By Keith Tindall from White Egret Farm. Used by permission.

EASY BROILED STEAK

1 sirloin or porterhouse steak	Butter

Broil steak under hot flame or in hot frying pan, turning frequently, until well browned. Place on serving dish and season as you like. You may add a pat of butter on top of the steak before serving. **SERVES 1.**
From *The Lazy Person's Whole Food Cookbook* by Stephen Byrnes. Used by permission.

EASY LAMB STEW

1½ lb. lamb stew meat	1½ cups diced potatoes
1½ cups diced carrots	¼ cup chopped onion
1 cup diced celery	1 tsp. Celtic sea salt
¼ Cup canned tomatoes	

Brown the lamb in extra-virgin coconut oil. Cover with water and add salt. Simmer until meat is tender. Add vegetables and cover. Simmer for 30 minutes or until vegetables are cooked.
    This recipe can be made in a Crock-Pot and left to cook for the whole day. Simply add all your ingredients to the pot, cover, and switch on. **SERVES 6.**
From *The Lazy Person's Whole Food Cookbook* by Stephen Byrnes. Used by permission.

LAMB CHOPS

8 lamb chops	½ cup dry red wine
Freshly ground pepper	2 to 3 cups beef or lamb stock

You will need a very well-seasoned cast-iron skillet for this recipe. Season the lamb chops with pepper and cut off any excess fat. Place the skillet over a moderately high fire. When it is hot, set four chops in the pan. (No fat is required. The lamb chops will render their own fat, enough to keep the chops from sticking.) Cook about 5 minutes until they are rare or medium rare. Keep in a warm oven while you are cooking the second batch and preparing the sauce.

Pour the grease out of the pan and deglaze with the red wine and the beef stock. Boil rapidly, skimming off any dirty foam that rises to the top. Reduce to about 3/4 cup. The sauce should be consistency of maple syrup.

Place the lamb chops on heated plates, with their accompanying vegetables, and spoon on the sauce. **SERVES 4.**

From *Nourishing Traditions* by Sally Fallon. Used by permission.

LEG OF LAMB OR CHEVON

1 6–8 lb. leg of lamb or chevon (goat), pasture fed preferred	1 clove garlic, slivered
½ cup Dijon mustard	1-inch piece of ginger, skinned and minced
1 Tbsp. rosemary, fresh and finely minced	2 Tbsp. olive oil

Preheat the oven to 350 degrees. Blend mustard, soy sauce, herbs, and ginger in a bowl. Beat in oil to make a creamy mixture. Make 4 shallow slashes in the meat with a sharp knife; tuck a sliver of garlic into each. Brush the lamb or goat liberally with the sauce and let stand for 1–2 hours. Roast on a rack for 1¼ to 1 ½ hours, or until a meat thermometer reads 150 degrees. This will produce a medium degree of doneness. Allow to rest before carving. The temperature will climb to about 160 degrees as the meat rests. **SERVES 4–6.**

By Keith Tindall from White Egret Farm. Used by permission.

EASY PEPPER STEAK

4 equal-sized pieces of steak (sirloin or top round), about 1 inch thick	1 large red onion, chopped into 4 slices
	Olive oil
1 egg, beaten and diluted with a little water	Sea salt and pepper to taste
1 red or yellow pepper, seeded and chopped into 4 slices	Soy sauce

Place steak in a large bowl and add the egg. Sprinkle with salt and pepper and let sit for 15 minutes. Match up the onion and pepper slices. In a shallow baking pan, place enough olive oil to cover the bottom. Place the four steaks in the pan and sprinkle a little soy sauce on top of each. Then place one onion and pepper slice on each. Place under the broiler for 3–4 minutes. When you turn the steaks, be sure to replace the pepper and onion slices back on the tops of the steaks. Cook for another 3–4 minutes. **SERVES 4.**

From *The Lazy Person's Whole Food Cookbook* by Stephen Byrnes. Used by permission.

SIMPLE BEEF BURGUNDY

2 lb. lean beef stew meat in small cubes (preferably from pasture-fed beef)	1 cup burgundy wine
2 Tbsp. whole-grain flour (soaked overnight)	1 medium onion, chopped
2 Tbsp. butter	2 carrots, sliced
1 Tbsp. olive oil	8 oz. Crimini mushrooms, sliced
1 tsp. sea salt or Herbamare	1 clove garlic, minced
¼ tsp. pepper	1 bay leaf
2 cups brown beef stock (page 231)	¼ tsp. ground thyme
	1 Tbsp. parsley, snipped

Toss the meat in the flour, salt, and pepper in a brown paper bag. Remove. Brown in the butter/olive oil combination. Add the beef stock, wine, mushrooms, onion, carrots, garlic, bay leaf, and thyme. Simmer 2½ to 3 hours, until the meat is tender. Turn the burner off and add the parsley to the hot mixture. If more liquid is needed during cooking, add more stock and wine in proportions of 2 parts stock to 1 part wine. **SERVES 4–6.**

By Keith Tindall from White Egret Farm. Used by permission.

FAMILY ROAST BEEF

4–5 lb. chuck roast, preferably from grass-fed beef	½ cup Worcestershire sauce
¼ pound butter	Celtic sea salt
	Black pepper, freshly ground

Preheat oven to 325 degrees. Rub the roast with salt and pepper and place in a baking dish with 2-inch sides. In a saucepan, melt the butter and add an equal volume of Worcestershire sauce. Pour the sauce over the roast. Bake slowly at 325 degrees until a meat thermometer reads 150–155 degrees (for medium). Remove the roast from the oven and allow it to rest and redistribute the juices before carving. The temperature will climb to 160 degrees. It is particularly important that grass-fed beef be cooked more slowly at a lower temperature than commercial beef. Grass-fed beef should also be allowed to "coast in" to the desired level of doneness by removing it from the oven several minutes before you think it is done. This preserves the juiciness and produces meat that is tenderer.

NOTE: Worcestershire sauce was originally based on lacto-fermented green English walnut catsup (in addition to the fish pastes).

By Keith Tindall from White Egret Farm. Used by permission.

FRENCH-STYLE LONDON BROIL

1 or 2 flank steaks (preferably from pasture-fed beef)	2 Tbsp. onion, minced
½ cup olive oil	1 clove garlic, minced
½ cup burgundy wine	1½ tsp. salt
	5 drops of Tabasco sauce

Score both sides of the steaks in a diamond pattern about 18 inch deep. Combine all the ingredients in a large shallow baking dish. Coat the steaks with the marinade and turn four times during a 2-hour period of marinating in the refrigerator. (You may also marinate overnight.) Remove the steaks from the marinade and broil for 3–5 minutes on each side. To serve, cut diagonally into thin slices. **SERVES 3–4.**

By Keith Tindall from White Egret Farm. Used by permission.

KOREAN BEEF

1 flank steak	6 cloves garlic, peeled and mashed
½ cup soy sauce	2 Tbsp. sesame seeds
2 Tbsp. toasted sesame oil	¼ tsp. cayenne pepper
1 bunch green onions, finely chopped	

Using a very sharp and heavy knife, slice the flank steak as thinly as possible across the grain and on the diagonal. (This will be easier if the meat is partially frozen.) Mix other ingredients and marinate beef in the mixture, refrigerated, for several hours or overnight.

Fold or "ribbon" the strips and stick them on skewers, making 4 to 6 brochettes. Cook on barbecue or under grill, about 5 to 7 minutes per side. Meat should still be rare or medium rare inside. This is delicious with any fermented vegetables, especially ginger carrots. The lactic-acid-producing bacteria in the fermented vegetables are the perfect antidote to carcinogens that may have formed in the meat, especially if it has been barbecued. **SERVES 4.**

From *Nourishing Traditions* by Sally Fallon. Used by permission.

VENISON STEAKS WITH MARINADE

4–6 venison steaks, ½ inch thick	3 or 4 juniper berries
1 Tbsp. butter	1 sprig parsley
2 Tbsp. sesame oil	1 sprig thyme
	2 bay leaves
MARINADE:	1–2 cloves garlic, crushed
1 cup red wine	1 pinch of nutmeg
¼ cup lemon juice	1 tsp. sea salt or Herbamare
½ cup olive oil	1 dash hot pepper sauce

Combine the ingredients in the marinade. Marinate the steaks for 24 hours in the refrigerator. To keep the steaks juicy on the inside but brown on the outside, sauté 5–6 minutes on a side in the butter/sesame oil combination. **SERVES 4–6.**

By Keith Tindall from White Egret Farm. Used by permission.

ORGAN MEATS

Preparation Tip: Try to marinate organ meats for about 2 hours prior to cooking as it will significantly improve the taste. Place meat in container, cover with water, and then add 1–2 Tbsp. of fresh lemon juice, plain yogurt, or raw apple cider vinegar. Cover and place in refrigerator. When ready to cook, pour off water and rinse meat under cold water.

LIVER WITH TURKEY BACON AND ONIONS

1–2 lb. organic beef liver	1 egg, beaten
8 pieces of turkey bacon	½ cup whole-grain flour (soaked overnight)
1 onion, chopped	

Marinate the liver before cooking. Wash and dry the liver slices and set aside on a plate. Fry the bacon till crisp in a large skillet or frying pan. Remove bacon from the pan. Dredge the liver slices first in the egg, then in the flour. Place in a skillet and cook in extra-virgin coconut oil or butter.

The pieces will cook quickly, so be sure to turn after 2–3 minutes. (Don't overcook liver; it tastes terrible.) Melt some butter in another skillet and sauté onions in it. Strew the onions over the liver on a large platter and top with crumbled turkey bacon. **SERVES 4–6.**

Note: You can prepare this recipe without the turkey bacon, sautéing the liver in butter or extra-virgin coconut oil instead and serve with onions only.

From *The Lazy Person's Whole Food Cookbook* by Stephen Byrnes. Used by permission.

LIVER, RICE CASSEROLE

1 lb. chopped cooked liver	1 cup boiling water
3 Tbsp. melted butter	1 onion, chopped and sautéed in butter
2 cups cooked brown rice	Herbamare seasoning to taste
2 cups chopped tomatoes (you may use canned)	

Grease your casserole dish. Place onions on the bottom, then liver, then the rice. Add tomatoes, water, and seasoning. Bake at 400 degrees for 20 minutes. **SERVES 6.**

From *The Lazy Person's Whole Food Cookbook* by Stephen Byrnes. Used by permission.

GRAINS, NUTS, SEEDS, AND LEGUMES

PREPARATION TIPS

FOR WHOLE GRAINS: For millet, brown rice, oatmeal, amaranth, etc., soak desired amount of grain in an equal amount of water to which you've added 1 Tbsp. raw vinegar, fresh lemon juice, or plain yogurt. (Use 2–3 Tbsp. if you're cooking a large amount of grain.) Cover and let sit at room temperature for at least 7 hours, preferably longer. When ready to cook, add remaining required amount of water or stock and cook. NOTE: To soak whole-grain flours or pancake mixes, follow the same procedure as above but make sure the flour is mixed well with the soaking water.

FOR RAW BEANS AND LENTILS: Soak desired amount of beans in an equal amount of water to which you've added 1 Tbsp. raw vinegar, fresh lemon juice, or plain yogurt. (Use 2–3 Tbsp. if you're cooking a large amount of beans or lentils.) Cover and let sit at room temperature for at least 7 hours, preferably longer. When ready to cook, discard soaking water; add remaining required amount of water or stock and cook.

FOR RAW NUTS AND SEEDS: Place raw nuts or seeds in a bowl, add 1 Tbsp. sea salt, and cover with water. Leave at room temperature for 6–8 hours. Drain the water. Place nuts on a cookie sheet and dry on low heat in the oven. You can also air-dry the nuts on a towel, but it takes much longer to dry them this way.

SPROUTED ALMONDS

Sprouted almonds are much more digestible than untreated ones. Rinse 3 times per day. Ready in 3 days. Sprout is merely a tiny white appendage, about ⅛-inch long.

From *Nourishing Traditions* by Sally Fallon. Used by permission.

BREAKFAST PORRIDGE

1 cup oats, steel cut or rolled, or coarsely ground in your own grinder 1 cup water plus 2 Tbsp. fermented whey, yogurt, or buttermilk	½ tsp. Celtic sea salt 1 cup water 1 Tbsp. flaxseeds (optional)

For highest benefits and best assimilation, porridge should be soaked overnight or even longer. (Ancient recipes from Wales and Brittany called for a 24-hour soaking.) Once soaked, oatmeal cooks up in less than 5 minutes—truly a fast food.

Mix oats and salt with water mixture; cover and let stand at room temperature for at least 7 hours and as long as 24 hours. Bring additional 1 cup of water to boil. Add soaked oats. Reduce heat, cover, and simmer several minutes. Meanwhile, grind flaxseeds in a mini-grinder. Off heat, stir in flaxseeds and let stand for a few minutes. Serve with butter or cream thinned with a little water, and a natural sweetener like Sucanat, date sugar, maple syrup, or raw honey. **SERVES 4.**

From *Nourishing Traditions* by Sally Fallon. Used by permission.

CRISPY PECANS

4 cups pecan halves 1 tsp. sea salt or Herbamare	Filtered water

The buttery flavor of pecans is enhanced by soaking and slow-oven drying. Soak pecans in salt and filtered water for at least 7 hours or overnight. Drain in a colander. Spread pecans on two stainless steel baking pans and place in a warm oven (no more than 150 degrees) for 12 to 24 hours, stirring occasionally, until completely dry and crisp. Store in an airtight container. Great for school lunches. **MAKES 4 CUPS.**

VARIATION: TAMARI PECANS

In place of salt, add ¼ cup tamari sauce to soaking water.

From *Nourishing Traditions* by Sally Fallon. Used by permission.

EASY BROWN RICE

2 cups brown rice 4 cups water or 2 cups water mixed with 2 cups chicken stock	1 Tbsp. apple cider vinegar or yogurt

Soak rice in 2 cups of water with the vinegar or yogurt for at least 7 hours. Transfer to your pot or rice cooker. Add the remaining water or water/broth, and cook till tender. If you're cooking the rice on a stovetop, bring to a boil then lower heat to a simmer and cook covered, stirring occasionally. **SERVES 6–8.**
NOTE: This recipe can be used for ANY whole grain you wish to serve by itself—millet, quinoa, buckwheat, amaranth, etc.
From *The Lazy Person's Whole Food Cookbook* by Stephen Byrnes. Used by permission.

EASY FRENCH TOAST

1 cup plain yogurt ½ tsp. honey 2 eggs, slightly beaten	½ tsp. sea salt 8 slices sprouted or sourdough whole-grain bread

Combine eggs, yogurt, honey, and salt in a mixing bowl. Dip each slice of bread quickly into the mixture. Brown in extra-virgin coconut oil. Serve with butter and unheated honey or maple syrup or fresh fruit. **SERVES 4.**
From *The Lazy Person's Whole Food Cookbook* by Stephen Byrnes. Used by permission.

EASY WHOLE-GRAIN WAFFLES

1⅓ cups whole-grain flour (spelt, kamut) ¾ tsp. sea salt 2 tsp. non-aluminum baking powder 2 Tbsp. unheated honey	1 cup water 2 Tbsp. plain yogurt 4 Tbsp. extra-virgin coconut oil 2 eggs, separated

Soak the flour in water with 2 Tbsp. yogurt for at least 7 hours. Separate the eggs. Beat the yolks and add the yogurt and butter. Combine salt, honey, and flour; add this to the first mixture. Beat the egg whites until they form stiff peaks; fold them into the mix. Mix in the baking powder quickly. Cook in your waffle iron. **SERVES 6.**
From *The Lazy Person's Whole Food Cookbook* by Stephen Byrnes. Used by permission.

FIVE-GRAIN CEREAL MIX

2 cups wheat or spelt 2 cups millet 2 cups short-grain rice	2 cups barley or oats 2 cups split peas or lentils

This combination of grains conforms to the five grains recommended in the *Yellow Emperor's Classic of Internal Medicine*. Mix together and grind coarsely. Store in refrigerator. **MAKES 10 CUPS.**
From *Nourishing Traditions* by Sally Fallon. Used by permission.

FIVE-GRAIN PORRIDGE

1 cup Five-Grain Cereal 1 cup water plus 2 Tbsp. fermented whey or yogurt	½ tsp. Celtic sea salt 1 cup water 1 Tbsp. flaxseeds (optional)

Mix Five-Grain Cereal and salt with water plus whey or yogurt. Cover and let stand at room temperature for at least 7 hours and as long as 24 hours. Bring additional 1 cup of water to boil. Add soaked cereal. Reduce heat, cover, and simmer several minutes. Meanwhile, grind flaxseed in a mini-grinder. Remove cereal from heat and stir in flaxseed. Serve with butter or cream, thinned with a little water, and a natural sweetener like Sucanat, date sugar, maple syrup, or raw honey. **SERVES 4.**
From *Nourishing Traditions* by Sally Fallon. Used by permission.

MUFFINS

1¼ cups freshly ground and/or soaked spelt, kamut, or whole-wheat flour ¾ cup water mixed with 1 Tbsp. yogurt 1 egg, lightly beaten ¼ tsp. fine Celtic sea salt	½ cup extra-virgin coconut oil ⅓ cup honey 2 tsp. baking powder 1 tsp. vanilla

Preheat oven to 400 degrees. Mix flour with water and yogurt and let stand overnight. Mix in remaining ingredients. Pour into well-buttered muffin tin about three-quarters full. Bake for 15–20 minutes. These muffins will puff up and then fall back a bit to form flat tops. Note: 1 cup buckwheat flour or cornmeal may be used in place of 1 cup spelt, kamut, or wheat flour. **MAKES ABOUT 12.**

Adapted from *Nourishing Traditions* by Sally Fallon. Used by permission.

VARIATION: RAISIN MUFFINS
Add ½ cup raisins and ½ tsp. cinnamon to batter.

VARIATION: BLUEBERRY MUFFINS
Pour batter into muffin tins. Place 5–7 blueberries, fresh or frozen, on each muffin. Berries will fall into the muffins. (If they are added to the batter, they sink to the bottom of the muffin.)

VARIATION: DRIED CHERRY MUFFINS
Add 4 oz. dried cherries (available at health food stores and gourmet markets) and ½ cup chopped crispy pecans to batter.

VARIATION: FRUIT SPICE MUFFINS
Add 2 ripe pears or peaches, peeled and cut into small pieces, and ½ tsp. cinnamon, ⅛ tsp. cloves, and ⅛ tsp. nutmeg to batter.

VARIATION: LEMON MUFFINS
Add grated rind of 2 lemons and ½ cup chopped crispy pecans to batter. Omit vanilla.

VARIATION: GINGER MUFFINS
Add 1 Tbsp. freshly grated ginger and 1 tsp. ground ginger to batter. Omit vanilla.

BLUEBERRY PECAN PANCAKES

1½ cups freshly ground or soaked spelt, kamut, or whole-wheat flour ¾ cup water mixed with 1 Tbsp. yogurt 1 egg, lightly beaten ½ cup blueberries (fresh or frozen)	½ cup crispy pecans ¼ tsp. fine Celtic sea salt ½ cup extra-virgin coconut oil 2 tsp. baking powder 1 tsp. vanilla

Mix flour with water and yogurt and let stand overnight. Defrost blueberries in refrigerator if frozen. Mix ingredients into a bowl. Heat extra-virgin coconut oil in a skillet or pan over low heat. Increase temperature to moderate heat. Use about 3 Tbsp. of batter for each pancake. Serve with honey, maple syrup, or butter. **MAKES ABOUT 12.**

VARIATIONS: Use different kinds of fruit.

From *Nourishing Traditions* by Sally Fallon. Used by permission.

PEPITAS

4 cups raw, hulled pumpkin seeds 1 Tbsp. sea salt or Herbamare	1 tsp. cayenne pepper (optional) Filtered water

This recipe imitates Aztec practices of soaking seeds in brine, then letting them dry in the hot sun. They ate pepitas whole or ground into meal.

Dissolve salt in water and add pumpkin seeds and optional cayenne. Soak for at least 7 hours or overnight. Drain in a colander, then spread on 2 stainless steel baking pans. Place in a warm oven (no more than 150 degrees) for about 12 hours or overnight, stirring occasionally, until thoroughly dry and crisp. Store in an airtight container. **MAKES 4 CUPS.**

VARIATION: TAMARI PEPITAS Use 2 Tbsp. tamari sauce in place of sea salt and cayenne.

From *Nourishing Traditions* by Sally Fallon. Used by permission.

SIMPLE BEANS

2 cups black beans, kidney beans, pinto beans, black-eyed beans, or white beans Filtered water	2 Tbsp. whey 1 tsp. sea salt 4 cloves garlic, peeled and mashed (optional)

Soak beans in filtered water, salt, and whey for 12–24 hours, depending on the size of the bean. Drain, rinse, place in a large pot, and add water to cover beans. Bring to a boil, skimming off foam. Reduce heat and add optional garlic. Simmer, covered, for 4–8 hours. Check occasionally and add more water as necessary. **SERVES 8.**

From *Nourishing Traditions* by Sally Fallon. Used by permission.

SIMPLE LENTILS

2 cups lentils, preferably green lentils Filtered water 2 Tbsp. homemade whey or yogurt 1 tsp. Celtic sea salt 2 cups beef or chicken stock	2 cloves garlic, peeled and mashed Several sprigs fresh thyme, tied together 1 tsp. dried peppercorns, crushed Pinch dried chili flakes (optional) Juice of 1–2 lemons

Soak lentils in filtered water, salt, and whey for several hours. Drain and rinse. Place in a pot and add stock to cover. Bring to a boil and skim. Add remaining ingredients except lemon and simmer, uncovered, for about 1 hour, or until liquid has completely reduced. Add lemon juice and season to taste. Serve with a slotted spoon. Excellent with sauerkraut and strongly flavored meats such as duck, game, or lamb. **SERVES 6–8.**

From *Nourishing Traditions* by Sally Fallon. Used by permission.

SPROUTED SUNFLOWER SEEDS

These are among the most satisfactory seeds for sprouting. Sunflower sprouts are just delicious in salads, but they must be eaten very soon after sprouting is accomplished, as they soon go black. Try to find hulled sunflower seeds packed in nitrogen packs. Rinse 2 times per day. Ready in 12 to 18 hours, when sprout is just barely showing.

From *Nourishing Traditions* by Sally Fallon. Used by permission.

BEVERAGES

APPLE "CIDER"

1 gallon unfiltered, unpasteurized apple juice 1 Tbsp. sea salt	½ cup homemade whey

Place all ingredients in a large bowl. Cover and leave at room temperature for 2 days. Skim foam that rises to the top. Line a strainer with several layers of cheesecloth; strain juice into jars or jugs. Cover tightly and refrigerate. Flavors will develop slowly over several weeks. The "cider" will eventually develop a rich buttery taste.

If you wish to further clarify the cider, add lightly beaten egg whites to the jugs (1 egg white per quart). Set aside a few hours, and then filter again through several layers of cheesecloth. **MAKES 4 QUARTS.**

From *Nourishing Traditions* by Sally Fallon. Used by permission.

BALANCED VEGETABLE JUICE

Vegetable juices can be a great source of essential nutrients. Here is a staple vegetable juice blend:

50 percent carrot juice 10 percent beet juice 30 percent celery juice 10 percent parsley or other green juice	1 tsp. cream, goat's milk yogurt, coconut milk 1–2 Tbsp. of Green Superfood Powder with HSOs (optional)

By Jordan Rubin

CULTURED VEGETABLE JUICE

3 red beets	1 oz. grated ginger
1 carrot	1 tsp. fine Celtic sea salt
2–4 Tbsp. fermented whey or 1 packet cultured vegetable starter (see Appendix B)	Purified water

Peel and chop beets and carrot; combine with peeled and grated ginger. Place in a 1–2 quart glass container with a seal. Cover with water and add whey and salt. Stir well and cover. Leave at room temperature for 2–3 days, then transfer to the refrigerator.
By Jordan Rubin

GINGER ALE

¾ cup ginger, peeled and finely chopped or grated	2 tsp. Celtic sea salt
½ cup fresh lime juice	¼ cup homemade whey
¼–½ cup Rapadura or dehydrated cane juice	2 quarts filtered water

Place all ingredients in a 2-quart jug and fill with water. Stir well and cover tightly. Keep at room temperature for two days before transferring to the refrigerator. This will keep several months well chilled. To serve, strain and mix half ginger ale with half purified water or naturally sparkling water. Best consumed at room temperature, not cold. **MAKES 2 QUARTS.**
From *Nourishing Traditions* by Sally Fallon. Used by permission.

HOMEMADE KEFIR

1 qt. raw goat's or cow's milk	1 packet kefir starter (see Appendix B)

Pour into quart-size Mason jar. Add kefir starter. Set in a room temperature area for 12–48 hours, then transfer to refrigerator. A cupboard is an ideal place to ferment. The temperature range should be between 70–75 degrees. Kefir can last several months in the refrigerator and will become sourer over time.
By Jordan Rubin

NEW WINE

1 case organic concord, black, or red grapes, about 16 lb.	½ cup Probiogurt or continental acidophilus
	1 Tbsp. Celtic sea salt

This beverage is best made with a vegetable juicer, although a high-speed blender or food processor will do. It takes a bit of time, but the results are worth it. This delicious and refreshing drink is an excellent substitute for wine, containing all the nutrients of grapes found in wine, including many enzymes, but none of the alcohol. In fact, a drink similar to this may have been what the Bible referred to as "new wine."

Remove grapes from stems, wash well, and pass through the juicer. Place liquid in a large bowl with salt and Probiogurt, and stir well. Cover and leave at room temperature for 2 days. If you don't use a juicer, you may want to scoop off the skins and strain juice through a strainer lined with several layers of cheesecloth. It is best to store new wine in airtight containers in refrigerator. Delicious flavors will develop over time. May be served diluted with half water. **MAKES 5–6 QUARTS.**
By Jordan Rubin

RASPBERRY DRINK

2 12-oz. packages frozen raspberries, or 24 oz. fresh raspberries	¼ cup homemade whey
Juice of 12 oranges	2 tsp. Celtic sea salt
¼–½ cup Rapadura or dehydrated cane juice	2 quarts filtered water

Place raspberries in food processor and blend until smooth. Mix in a large bowl with remaining ingredients. Cover and let sit at room temperature for 2 days. Skim foam that may rise to top. Strain through a strainer lined with cheesecloth. Pour into jugs or jars. Cover tightly and store in refrigerator. If you wish to further clarify the raspberry drink, add lightly beaten egg whites to the jugs (1 egg white per quart). Set aside a few hours, and then filter again through several layers of cheesecloth. To serve, dilute with sparkling mineral water. **MAKES 2 QUARTS.**

From *Nourishing Traditions* by Sally Fallon. Used by permission.

SMOOTHIES

Author's note: During my healing process, I consumed this smoothie one to two times per day with raw eggs. Contrary to popular belief, eggs from healthy, free-range, pastured chickens are almost always free of dangerous germs. If the egg has an odor, obviously it should not be eaten. Since most of the salmonella infections are caused by germs on the shell, for added protection it is best to wash the eggs in the shell with a mild alcohol or hydrogen peroxide solution or a fruit and vegetable wash.

BERRY SMOOTHIE

10 oz. plain whole-milk yogurt, kefir, or coconut milk/cream 1–2 raw high omega-3 whole eggs (optional) 1 Tbsp. extra-virgin coconut oil	1 Tbsp. flaxseed or hempseed oil 1–2 Tbsp. unheated honey 1 Tbsp. goat's milk protein powder (optional) 1–2 cups fresh or frozen berries

Combine ingredients in a high-speed blender.

Properly prepared, this smoothie is an extraordinary source of easy-to-absorb nutrition. It contains large amounts of "live" enzymes, probiotics, vitally important "live" proteins, and a full spectrum of essential fatty acids. Smoothies should be consumed immediately or refrigerated for up to 24 hours. If frozen in ice cube trays with a toothpick inserted into each cube, smoothies can make for a great frozen dessert. **MAKES TWO 8-OZ. SERVINGS.**

By Jordan Rubin

VARIATIONS FOR SMOOTHIES

To enjoy the same life giving nutrients with different flavors, add the following ingredients to the "basic" ingredients used in the smoothie listed above:

BANANA COCONUT CREAM SMOOTHIE—10 oz. coconut milk/cream (instead of whole-milk yogurt or kefir); 1–2 fresh or frozen bananas (instead of berries); ½ tsp. vanilla extract

BLACKBERRY BANANA SMOOTHIE—½–1 cup fresh or frozen blackberries (instead of berries); 1 fresh or frozen banana

CHERRY VANILLA SMOOTHIE—½–1 cup fresh or frozen cherries (instead of berries); 1 fresh or frozen banana

CHOCOLATE MOUSSE SMOOTHIE—2 Tbsp. cocoa or carob powder or Healthy Chocolate Spread (instead of berries) (See Appendix B.)

CREAMSICLE SMOOTHIE—6 oz. (not 10) of plain whole-milk yogurt or kefir; 4 oz. freshly squeezed orange juice; 1–2 fresh or frozen bananas (instead of berries)

MOCHA SWISS ALMOND SMOOTHIE—2 Tbsp. cocoa or carob powder (instead of berries); 2 Tbsp. raw almond butter (or 4 Tbsp. Chocolate Almond Spread—see Appendix B)

MOCHACCINO SMOOTHIE—2 Tbsp. cocoa or carob powder; 1 Tbsp. organic-roasted coffee beans; 1–2 fresh or frozen bananas (instead of berries)

PEACHES 'N CREAM SMOOTHIE— ½–1 cup fresh or frozen peaches (instead of berries); 1 fresh or frozen banana

PINA COLADA SMOOTHIE—10 oz. coconut milk/cream (no whole-milk yogurt or kefir); 1 cup fresh or frozen pineapple (instead of berries); 1 fresh or frozen banana

By Jordan Rubin

SNACKS AND DESSERTS

BANANA BREAD

3 cups freshly ground spelt or wheat flour	¼ to ½ cup maple syrup
2 cups cultured buttermilk, water mixed with 2 Tbsp. whey or yogurt	2 tsp. baking soda
	¼ cup melted butter
3 eggs, lightly beaten	2 ripe bananas, mashed
1 tsp. sea salt	½ cup chopped crispy pecans

Mix flour with buttermilk or water mixture and let stand overnight. Beat in remaining ingredients. Pour into a well-buttered and floured loaf pan. Bake at 350 degrees for 1 hour or more, until a toothpick comes out clean. **MAKES ONE 9 X 13 LOAF.**
For variations of this recipe, order a copy of *Nourishing Traditions* by Sally Fallon. (See Appendix B.)

COCONUT ALMOND FUDGE

1 cup extra-virgin coconut oil	¼ cup unheated honey
¾ cup carob powder	1 Tbsp. vanilla
¼ cup raw almond butter	

Place all ingredients in a glass container and set in simmering water until melted if needed. Mix together well. Spread thick paste mixture on a piece of buttered parchment paper; allow to cool in refrigerator or freezer. Remove and serve immediately. **MAKES 1¼ CUP.**
By Jordan Rubin

PINEAPPLE CREAMY TREAT

1 cup organic ricotta cheese	½ tsp. vanilla extract
1 Tbsp. unheated honey	1 cup pineapple or fruit of choice

Mix ricotta, honey, and vanilla extract. Top with fruit of choice. **SERVES 2–3.**
By Jordan Rubin

CREAMY HIGH-ENZYME DESSERT

4 oz. Probiogurt, plain yogurt, or cultured cream	1 tsp. flaxseed oil
1 Tbsp. raw, unheated honey	½ cup fresh or frozen organic berries

Mix yogurt, honey, and flaxseed oil. Top with berries.
By Jordan Rubin

SUPER SEED BAR

¾ cup and 3 Tbsp. SuperSeed Whole Food Fiber Powder (See Appendix B.)	6 Tbsp. cocoa or carob powder
½ cup tahini (sesame butter)	¼ tsp. salt
½ cup almond butter	1/3 cup honey
¼ cup and 1 Tbsp. Goatein goat's milk protein powder (See Appendix B.)	2½ Tbsp. extra-virgin coconut oil
	1 tsp. vanilla extract
	1 tsp. orange or almond extract

Combine wet and dry ingredients and form into bars. Freeze or refrigerate. **MAKES 4–6 3-OZ. BARS.**
By Phyllis Rubin. Used by permission.
VARIATIONS Add organic chocolate or carob chips, shredded coconut, dried fruit, or chopped almonds.

TRAIL MIX

1 cup crispy pecans	1 cup raisins
1 cup crispy cashews	1 cup dried sweetened coconut meat
1 cup unsulphured dried apricots, apples, pears, or pineapple cut into pieces	1 cup carob chips (optional)

Mix all ingredients together. Store in an airtight container. **MAKES 5–6 CUPS.**

From *Nourishing Traditions* by Sally Fallon. Used by permission.

ZESTY POPCORN

⅓ cup popcorn	2 Tbsp. melted butter
3 Tbsp. extra-virgin coconut oil	Herbamare to taste
2 Tbsp. garlic-chili flax	

Melt coconut oil in pan over medium heat. Pour popcorn into pan. Cover pan with lid. While popping, melt butter. Cook until popped. Pour into large bowl. Pour melted butter and garlic chili-flax and seasoning and mix thoroughly.

By Nicki Rubin. Used by permission.

Acknowledgments

MANY PEOPLE SAY THAT WRITING A BOOK IS MUCH LIKE HAVING AND raising a baby. It starts as a concept, then it becomes a dream, and then it begins to feel like a chore. Later you wonder how you could ever have been entrusted with something so great, so important.

Soon you have questions like "How in the world will I ever get this right? How did I get myself into this in the first place?"

No matter what goes through your mind during the process, whenever you think about it, you feel joy, excitement, wonder, and a huge sense of awe and responsibility—emotions that I felt when I was writing this book and Nicki and I were expecting our first child.

Once again, I am asking some of the same questions. One thing I know for sure, when God births something in you—an idea, a dream, or even a child— He will take full responsibility to make it everything He wants it to be if you will just let Him.

Many people have helped me birth and raise this book. I would first like to thank my beautiful wife, Nicki, who made me believe that I could do anything with God's help. I also want to thank the following:

* My mother and father, who taught me the principles of natural health and led me to a relationship with God.
* My Grandma Rose, who told me that everything I do is worthy of a Nobel prize.
* My sister, Jenna, who witnessed firsthand my journey from sickness to health and prayed for me the entire time.

- Larry Walker, who helped turn this idea into a reality.
- Two of my best friends and colleagues, Jason Dewberry and Kenny Duke, who told me more than twenty years ago when I was living in an RV by the beach in San Diego that they wanted to be a part of my future—and they were.
- Mike and Meredith Berkich, who have constantly encouraged me to be all that God wants me to be.
- Dr. Charles Stanley, who told me that God has big plans for my life and that this message of health and hope will change the lives of millions.
- Christian music artist Michael Neale, who helped me turn some words on a page into a great song.
- Dr. Peter Rothschild, who has taught me many things about health and gave me the name of this book
- William "Bud" Keith, who pointed me to the greatest health book of all time, the Bible.

Most importantly, I want to give thanks to a loving and compassionate God who looked down from heaven, found a 100-pound, six-foot-tall lump of clay, and fashioned me into His handiwork.

May I serve You all the rest of my days.

Source Material

Introduction

"Today, two-thirds of American adults are overweight, and one of three adults are obese…" is from "Overweight and Obesity Statistics," National Institutes for Health, and available at https://www.niddk.nih.gov/health-information/health-statistics/overweight-obesity

Chapter 1: From Tragedy to Triumph: My Personal Journey from Sickness to Health

"My father put me on an eating plan called the Specific Carbohydrate Diet, made popular by Elaine Gottschall, author of *Breaking the Vicious Cycle*, to help alleviate the thrush and the diarrhea…"

The premise of the Specific Carbohydrate Diet is that bacterial/fungal overgrowth causes damage to the intestinal walls in a vicious cycle that breaks down our health and immune systems. The goal of the diet is to eliminate certain carbohydrates containing sugars known as disaccharides (such as grains, sugar, dairy products, corn, and potatoes) that tend to nourish certain harmful bacteria and fungal species.

"With the sales of heartburn medications booming, some experts predict Crohn's disease may eventually surpass ulcers as the number one digestive problem in the United States" is from Digestive Disease Statistics, National Digestive Diseases Information Clearinghouse (NDDIC), a service of the National Institute of Diabetes and Digestive and Kidney Diseases and is http://digestive.niddk.nih.gov/statistics/statistics.htm.

"Dr. Morton Walker, a medical journalist who had supplied me information on some of the clinics I visited, asked if he could write an article outlining my amazing story…" is from "Homeostatic Soil Organisms for One's Primal Defense," by Morton Walker, DPM, *Townsend Letter for Doctors and Patients* (February/March 2001).

Chapter 2: The World's Healthiest People

"Elmer A. Josephson, a pioneer who dared to challenge the stream of
popular dietary trends, had this to say in his book, *God's Key to Health
and Happiness...*" is from *God's Key to Health and Happiness* by Elmer A.
Josephson, (Old Tappan, NJ: Fleming H. Revell Company, 1976), 160.

"The Top Five leading causes of hospitalizations..." is from "Distribution of
First-Listed Diagnoses Among Hospital Discharges with Diabetes as Any-
Listed Diagnoses, Adults Aged 18 Years and Older," by the Centers for
Disease Control and Prevention, 2010, and is available at http://www.cdc
.gov/diabetes/statistics/hosp/adulttable1.htm

"Peter Rothschild, M.D., Ph.D., wrote an unpublished book entitled *The Art
of Health*. In a chapter called "Please Don't Eat the Wrapper," he had this
to say..." is from an unpublished book entitled *The Art of Health* by Peter
Rothschild, M.D., Ph.D.

"The Hebrew words used to describe "unclean meats" can be translated as "foul,
polluted, and putrid..." is from "Strong's Electronic Concordance (KJV)," s.v.
"*tame.*" Copyright © 1989, TriStar Publishing. All rights reserved.

"The late Elmer Josephson was a pastor, missionary, and cancer survivor. In his
landmark volume *God's Key to Health and Happiness*, he wrote..." is from
God's Key to Health and Happiness by Elmer A. Josephson, (Old Tappan, NJ:
Fleming H. Revell Company, 1976), 47.

"Josephson claimed the pig's single stomach arrangement was very simple in
design and function in keeping with a limited excretory organ system..." is
from Ibid, 46.

"As the plague continued its scourge, it became apparent that the Jewish people
were somehow escaping its death grip..." is from *The Word on Health: A
Biblical and Medical* by Dr. Michael D. Jacobson, (Chicago: Moody Press,
2000), 11.

"The title of the study says it all: 'Apparent Absence of Stroke and Ischaemic
Heart Disease'..." is from "Apparent Absence of Stroke and Ischaemic Heart
Disease in a Traditional Melanesian Island: A Clinical Study of Kitava," by S.
Lindeberg and B. Lundh, *J Intern Med* 233 (1993): 269–275.

"Michael Murray, N.D., has written extensively about the absence of modern
disease from primitive cultures..." is from *Encyclopedia of Natural Medicine*
by M. Murray and J. Pizzorno, (Rocklin, CA: Prima Publishing, 1998).

"More than a century ago, in 1913, the Nobel Prize-winning physician and
missionary Albert Schweitzer visited Gabon, Africa, and had this to say..." is
from *Cancer: Cause and Cure*, Albert Schweitzer, in his preface to A. Berglas,

as quoted in James South, MA, "Laetrile—the Answer to Cancer," IAS
   Bulletin, http://www.antiaging-systems.com/extract/laetrile.htm
"Explorer and anthropologist Vilhjalmur Stefansson searched in vain for cases
   of cancer..." is from *Cancer: Disease of Civilization* by Vilhjalmur Stefanson,
   (New York: Hill and Wang, 1960).
"Kerin O'Dea, a professor at Monash University in Clayton, Victoria, attributes
   the diabetes increase to dietary changes..." is from "Marked Improvement
   in Carbohydrate and Lipid Metabolism in Diabetic Australian Aborigines
   After Temporary Reversion to Traditional Lifestyle," by K. O'Dea, *Lipids* 33
   (1984): 596–603.
"Dr. Price reported his findings in the book that he aptly titled, *Nutrition and
   Physical Degeneration*..." is from *Nutrition and Physical Degeneration*, by
   Weston Price, sixth ed. (Los Angeles: Price-Pottenger Foundation, 1939,
   1997).
"This was abundantly clear at a North American research site in the Illinois
   Valley..." is from "The Lower Illinois River Region: A Prehistoric Context for
   the Study of Ancient Diet and Health," by J. E. Buikstra in M. N. Cohen and
   G. J. Armelagos, eds., *Paleopathology at the Origins of Agriculture* (Orlando,
   FL: Academic Press), 217–230.
"Compared to the appearance of these first people at the Dickson Mounds, there
   was a general increase in the reliance on maize or corn..." is from "Health
   Changes at Dickson Mounds, Illinois" by A. H. Goodman, et al., in Cohen
   and Armelagos, *Paleopathology at the Origins of Agriculture*, 271–305.
"The *Palm Beach Post* article had this to say..." is from "China's Taste for Critters
   May Have Aided SARS," by Michael Browning, *Palm Beach Post*, May 25,
   2003.

Chapter 3: Life and Death in a Long Hollow Tube: The Importance of the GI Tract

"Regarding the latter, 40 percent of Americans who die each year..." is from
   "Up to 40 percent of annual deaths from each of the five leading US causes
   are preventable" by the Centers for Disease Control and Prevention, and is
   available at: http://www.cdc.gov/media/releases/2014/p0501-preventable
   -deaths.html
"The Merriam-Webster dictionary defines gut as..." comes from the Merriam-
   Webster Dictionary website and is available at http://www.merriam-webster
   .com/dictionary/gut
"Award-winning science writer Sandra Blakeslee specializes in "cognitive
   neuroscience..." is from "Complex and Hidden Brain in Gut Makes

Stomachaches and Butterflies," by Sandra Blakeslee, *New York Times*, January 23, 1996.

"Dr. Michael Gershon, chairman of the department of anatomy and cell biology at Columbia University in New York City, has devoted his career to understanding the human bowel..." is from *The Second Brain* by Dr. Michael Gershon, (New York: HarperCollins, 1998).

"Dr. Michael Loes, a pain management specialist and author of *The Healing Response*..." is from *The Healing Response* by Michael Loes, M.D., M.D. (Freedom Press, 2002).

"Dr. H. H. Boeker, who studied the digestive tract, stated in 1928..." is from "Autointoxication," by H. H. Boeker, *Medical Journal and Record* 128 (September 19, 1928): 293.

Chapter 4: Hygiene: The Double-Edged Sword

"History records that the Egyptians treated pinkeye with "the urine of a faithful wife" and favored other treatments..." is from *None of These Diseases* by S. I. McMillen, M.D. and David E. Stern, M.D., (Grand Rapids, MI: Fleming H. Revell, 2000), 9–11, 13–14; citing excerpts from *The Edwin Smith Surgical Papyrus*, trans. James H. Breasted (Chicago: University of Chicago Press, 1930), 473–475.

"In the eighteenth century, London's chimney sweeps had an extraordinarily high rate of scrotal cancer... " is *Why the Need for Better Hygiene*, by Kenneth Seaton, Ph.D., and available at www.advancedhygieneproducts.com/why _the _need_for_better_hygiene.shtml.

"More than 60 million Americans—one in every five—suffer from allergies or have an asthma infection..." from "Allergy Facts and Figures," Asthma and Allergy Foundation of America, and available at http://www.aafa.org/display .cfm?id=9&sub=30

"Consider these alarm bells sounded by the folks at *Consumer Reports* in 2014..." from "Antibiotics are becoming less effective, and their overuse is making them dangerous," by *Consumer Reports* and published on the *Washington Post* website at http://goo.gl/VyVrLU.

"Many current antibiotics come from microbes in the soil, including streptomycin, the first treatment for tuberculosis..." is from "Down in the Dirt, Wonders Beckon: Soil and Sea Yield Unknown Lodes of Useful Microbes," by P. Raeburn. *Business Week*, December 3, 2001.

"Twenty-five years ago, Dr. David Strachan, a respected epidemiologist at Britain's London School of Hygiene and Tropical Medicine..." is from "Let Them Eat Dirt," by M. Downey, *Toronto Star*, January 10, 1999, F1.

"Researchers estimate that by consuming just one glass of commercially processed and packaged milk from your local supermarket shelf…" is from *The Milk Book*, by William Campbell Douglass, M.D., revised ed. (Second Opinion Publishing, 1997).

"This dysbiosis, or bacterial imbalance in the gut, results in abnormal fermentation in the small intestine…" is from "Jejunal Bacterial Overgrowth and Intestinal Permeability in Children With Immunodeficiency Syndromes," by C. Pignata, et al., *Gut* 31 (1990): 879–882.

"Research has shown that the prevention and treatment of dysbiosis and dysbacteriosis are among the most challenging problems doctors face today…" is from "Problems in Drug Prevention and Treatment of Endogenous Infection and Dysbacteriosis," by V. M. Melfikova, et al., *Vestn Ross Akad Med Nauk* 3 (1997): 26–29.

"The following list briefly describes the health benefits that scientists attribute to the consumption of soil-based organisms…" is from "Medical Innovative Biologics: Homeostatic Soil Organisms Support Immune System Functions from the Ground Up," by M. Walter, *Townsend Letter for Doctors and Patients* (February/March 2001).

Chapter 5: How to Get Sick: A Modern Prescription for Illness

"Rex Russell, M.D., noted that when sunlight activates the phytochemicals in healthy foods…" is from *What the Bible Says About Healthy Living* by Rex Russell, M.D., Revell, 2006, pg. 241.

"A study published in *The Lancet* (a respected medical journal in Great Britain) indicated that chronic sleep loss…" is from *Lancet* 354 (October 23, 1999): 1435–1439.

"For more information about these products and possible alternative choices, see *The Safe Shopper's Bible*…" is from *The Safe Shopper's Bible: A Consumer's Guide to Nontoxic Household Products, Cosmetics, and Food* by David Steinman and Samuel S. Epstein, M.D., (New York: Hungry Minds, Inc., 1995), 265–266, 355, 427, 434.

"A top EPA scientific advisor voiced the opinion…" is from *Diet for a Poisoned Planet: How to Choose Safe Foods for You and Your Family* by David Steinman (New York: Harmony Books, a division of Crown Publishers, 1990), 225–226.

"Renowned diabetes expert Dr. H. J. Roberts believes there is a clear scientific link between aspartame and increased incidence of brain tumors…" is from *Aspartame (NutraSweet): Is It Safe?* by Dr. H. J. Roberts, (Philadelphia: The Charles Press, Publishers, September 1992).

"Excessive showering—even in the purest water—can rob your hair and body of natural oils…" is from "Winter Brings Cold & Dry Itchy Skin," by Brian Bretsch, Barnes Jewish Hospital, and is available at http://www.barnesjewish.org/groups/default.asp?NavID+1014

"Studies show a strong link between chlorinated water supplies with elevated THM levels and cancers of the bladder, kidney, liver…" is from *Diet for a Poisoned Planet: How to Choose Safe Foods for You and Your Family* by David Steinman (New York: Harmony Books, a division of Crown Publishers, 1990), 208–209.

"Mother's milk is the Maker's perfect food for babies, delivered in the close bonds of maternal intimacy…" is from *What the Bible Says About Healthy Living* by Rex Russell, M.D., Revell, 2006, 215–216.

"San Diego State biology professor Scott Kelley took a small but scientific sampling of airline cleanliness…" is from "Molecular Survey of Aeroplane Bacterial Contamination," by C. J. McManus and S. T. Kelley, *Journal of Applied Microbiology* 99 (3) (2005), 502–508, doi: 10.1111/j.1365-2672.2005.02651.x.

"Everywhere you go, you run into electromagnetic fields (EMFs) from television sets, microwave ovens, cell phones…" is from *The Safe Shopper's Bible: A Consumer's Guide to Nontoxic Household Products, Cosmetics, and Food* by David Steinman and Samuel S. Epstein, M.D., (New York: Hungry Minds, Inc., 1995), 159.

"The organization cites one estimate that approximately '26 million amalgam bearers whose allergies may be causally related to their mercury/amalgam dental fillings'… " is from "BioProbe Frequently Asked Questions," and is available at http://www.bioprobe.com/faq.asp#top.

"My issue with contact lenses, especially the soft lens variety offered for long-term wear, is that they pose significant infection risks…" is from "Wearing Contacts Overnight Boosts Infection Risk," and is available at http://www.mercola.com/1999/archive/contacts_overnight_increase_infection.htm.

"Most pesticides are known carcinogens, and some of them pose as counterfeit versions of the female hormone estrogen…" is from *Toxic Relief* by Don Colbert, M.D., (Lake Mary, FL: Siloam, 2001), 16.

"… study by researchers at Johns Hopkins Medicine, medical errors are the third leading cause of death in the U.S.…." is from "Medical Errors Are No. 3 Cause of U.S. Deaths, Researchers Say," NPR Radio, by Marshall Allen and Olga Pierce, May 3, 2016, and available at https://www.npr.org/sections/health-shots/2016/05/03/476636183/death-certificates-undercount-toll-of-medical-errors.

Chapter 6: The Desperate Search for Health

"According to a National Institutes for Health survey released in 2015, U.S. adults are using alternative medicine methods 38 percent of the time…" is from "The Use of Complementary and Alternative Medicine in the United States," NIH National Center for Complementary and Integrative Health, and is available at https://nccih.nih.gov/research/statistics/2007/camsurvey_fs1.htm

"These nutritional deficiencies are nothing to sneeze at and pose potentially deadly consequences to long-term health…" is from "The Myths of Vegetarianism," by Stephen Byrnes, Ph.D., RNCP, *Townsend Letter for Doctors and Patients*, July 2000, revised January 2002.

"A comprehensive study of heart disease by Russell Smith…" is from *Diet, Blood Cholesterol and Coronary Heart Disease: A Critical Review of the Literature*, vol. 2 by Russell L. Smith, Ph.D., (N.p.: Vector Enterprises, 1991).

"Dr. Byrnes comments, 'If meat, fish, and eggs do indeed generate cancerous "ptyloamines," it is very strange'…" is from "The Myths of Vegetarianism," by Stephen Byrnes, Ph.D., RNCP, *Townsend Letter for Doctors and Patients*, July 2000, revised January 2002.

"For instance, the late Dr. Robert C. Atkins suggested that dieters treat themselves…" is from *Dr. Atkins' New Diet Revolution* by Robert Atkins, M.D., (New York: Avon Books, 1992), 280–281.

Chapter 7: Seven Victims Find Victory

"Positive research findings on the medicinal powers of mushrooms became prominent in research literature in the 1980s…" is from "Maitake D-fraction: Apoptosis Inducer and Immune Enhancer," by S. Konno, *Alternative and Complementary Therapies* (April 2001): 102–107.

"Several varieties—but not including the popular button mushroom from the grocery store—offer…" is from "Functional Properties of Edible Mushrooms," by R. Chang, *Nutr Rev* 54 (1996):S91–93.

Chapter 8: Return to the Maker's Diet

"The word protein is derived from the Greek word *proteus*, which literally means of primary importance…" is from Origin of the Word "Protein," *Protein and Amino Acids*, National Academy Press, http://books.nap.edu/books/0309063469/html/109.html

"If even one of these eight essential amino acids is missing, the body is unable to synthesize the other proteins it needs—no matter how much protein you eat…" is from *Nourishing Traditions: The Cookbook That Challenges Politically*

Correct Nutrition and the Diet Dictocrats, by Sally Fallon with Mary G. Enig, Ph.D., second ed. (Washington, DC: New Trends Publishing, Inc., 1999), 26.

"When your body fails to get the essential amino acids and protein it needs, you begin to lose myocardial (heart) muscle..." is from *Nourishing Traditions: The Cookbook That Challenges Politically Correct Nutrition and the Diet Dictocrats,* by Sally Fallon with Mary G. Enig, Ph.D., second ed. (Washington, DC: New Trends Publishing, Inc., 1999), 27, citing J. G. Webb, et al., *Canadian Medical Association Journal* 135 (October 1, 1986): 753–758.

"Studies show that soy protein isolates in such powders tend to be high in mineral-blocking phytates..." is from *Nourishing Traditions: The Cookbook That Challenges Politically Correct Nutrition and the Diet Dictocrats,* by Sally Fallon with Mary G. Enig, Ph.D., second ed. (Washington, DC: New Trends Publishing, Inc., 1999), 29, citing J. J. Rackis, et al., *Qual Plant Foods Hum Nutri* 35 (1985): 232.

"A study comparing Yemenite Jews in Israel who ate butter against those consuming margarine and vegetable oils yielded similar results..." is from "Soy Products for Dairy Products—Not So Fast," by Sally Fallon and Mary Enig, Ph.D., *Health Freedom News,* September 1995; citing M. DeBakey, et al., *JAMA* 189 (1964): 655–659; *Nutr Week* 21 (March 22, 1991): 2–3; A. Cohen, *Am Heart J* 65 (1963): 291.

"A list of the key roles of saturated fats is found in Nourishing Traditions, co-authored by Sally Fallon..." is from *Nourishing Traditions: The Cookbook That Challenges Politically Correct Nutrition and the Diet Dictocrats,* by Sally Fallon with Mary G. Enig, Ph.D., second ed. (Washington, DC: New Trends Publishing, Inc., 1999) 11.

"The authors summarize their study with this astounding statement..." is from Ibid., citing U. Ravnskov, *J Clin Epidemiol* 51 (June 1998): 443–460; C. V. Felton, et al., *Lancet* 344 (1994): 1195.

"Studies of African tribes have shown that intakes of enormous amounts of animal fat [do] not necessarily raise blood cholesterol..." is from *The Cholesterol Myths* by Uffe Ravnskov, M.D., Ph.D., (Washington, DC: New Trends Publishing, Inc., 2000), from an excerpt citing A. G. Shaper, "Cardiovascular Studies in the Samburu Tribe of Northern Kenya," *American Heart Journal* 63 (1962): 437–442, http://www.ravnskov.nu/myth3.htm

"Heart disease should be blamed not on animal fats or cholesterol..." is "Diet and Heart Disease—Not What You Think," by Sally Fallon with Mary G. Enig, Ph.D., *Consumer's Research,* July 1996, 15–19.

"Always shop for ocean-caught salmon—especially the varieties from cold Alaskan waters, which offer a healthful balance of omega-3 and omega-6 fatty acids..." is from *What the Bible Says About Healthy Living,* Rex Russell,

M.D., Revell, 2006, 148, citing Udo Erasmus, *Fats That Heal, Fats That Kill* (Burnaby, B.C., Canada: Alive Books, 1994), 232–233.

"The liberal consumption of omega-3 fatty acids is crucial for negating the effects of the overabundance of omega-6 linoleic acids…" is from *Nourishing Traditions: The Cookbook That Challenges Politically Correct Nutrition and the Diet Dictocrats*, by Sally Fallon with Mary G. Enig, Ph.D., second ed. (Washington, DC: New Trends Publishing, Inc., 1999) 29, citing Alfred J. Merrill, et al., *Ann Rev Nutr* 13 (1993): 539–559.

"Hydrogenated fats have been associated with cancer, atherosclerosis…" comes from *Trans Fatty Acids in the Food Supply: A Comprehensive Report Covering 60 Years of Research*, second ed., by Mary G. Enig, Ph.D., (Silver Spring, MD: Enig Associates, Inc., 1995); B. A. Watkins, et al., *Br Pouli Sci* 32 (December 1991): 1109–1119.

"Today, we gladly push aside healthier fare to gather fully one-fourth of our annual calorie intake from sugar—which is about 170 pounds of sugar each year…" is from *Nourishing Traditions: The Cookbook That Challenges Politically Correct Nutrition and the Diet Dictocrats*, by Sally Fallon with Mary G. Enig, Ph.D., second ed. (Washington, DC: New Trends Publishing, Inc., 1999), 23, citing Joseph D. Beasly, M.D., and Jerry J. Swift, M.A., *The Kellogg Report* (Annandale-on-Hudson, NY: The Institute of Health Policy and Practice, 1989), 144–145.

"When two United Nations agencies—the World Health Organization (WHO) and the Food and Agriculture Organization—released the results of a study…" is from CNN.com: "Global Health Group: Slash Sugar Intake—Experts Want No More Than 10 Percent of Calories From Sugar," March 3, 2003, and is available at http://edition.cnn.com/2003/HEALTH/diet .fitness/03/03/fat.world.ap

"And it directs the nation to consume even more carbohydrates from its USDA Food Guide Pyramid…" is from "Choose a Diet Moderate in Sugars," National Agricultural Library, USDA, and is available at http://www.nalusda .gov/fnic/dga/dga95/sugars.html.

"This is the same dietary picture and lifestyle that may put one out of every three Americans at risk of developing diabetes…" is from "One in Three Kids Will Develop Diabetes," citing "American Diabetes Association 63rd Scientific Sessions, New Orleans, June 13–17, 2003; K. M. Venkat Narayan, M.D., chief of the diabetes epidemiology section, CDC; Judith Fradkin, M.D., director of diabetes, endocrinology and metabolic diseases, NIDDK," and is available at http://my.webmd.com/content/Article/66/79851.htm.

"According to Fallon and Enig, "Studies show that these extruded whole grain preparations…" is from *Nourishing Traditions: The Cookbook That Challenges*

Politically Correct Nutrition and the Diet Dictocrats, by Sally Fallon with Mary G. Enig, Ph.D., second ed. (Washington, DC: New Trends Publishing, Inc., 1999), 25, citing David A. Jenkins, et al., *Am J Clin Nutr* 34 (March 1981): 362–366.

"The late Dr. Edward Howell…" for more information, read *Enzyme Nutrition* by Dr. Edward Howell, (Wayne, NJ: Avery Publishing Group, 1985).

"His later discovery of a primitive people who had almost no diabetes, constipation, or irritable bowel syndrome…" is from "Varicose Veins Among the Maasai?" by D. Burkitt, *Lancet* 1 (April 1973): 890.

"And according to Annelies Schoneck, author of *Making Sauerkraut and Pickled Vegetables at Home…*" is from *Des Crudites Toute L'Annee* by Annelies Schoneck from as cited in Sally Fallon in *Nourishing Traditions,* 93.

"Over 50 percent of the population take vitamin or mineral supplements to improve energy and performance…" is from "Consumer Research on Dietary Supplements," U.S. Food and Drug Administration, Center for Food Safety and Applied Nutrition, Consumer Studies Branch, http://vm.cfsan.fda.gov/~lrd/ab-suppl.html.

"He also discovered what he called Activator X…" is from "Ancient Dietary Wisdom for Tomorrow's Children," by Weston A. Price, The Weston A. Price Foundation, and is available at http://www.westonaprice.org/traditional_diets/ancient_dietary_wisdom.html.

"The higher the levels of omega-3 fatty acids in the blood, the lower your blood pressure and your risk of heart disease and cancer…" is from "Influence of Dietary Cod Liver Oil on Fatty Acid Composition of Plasma Lipids in Human Male Subjects After Myocardial Infarction," by G. V. Skuladottir, et al., *J Intern. Med* 228 (1990): 563–568.

"This has made cod liver oil a recommended first-response treatment for early symptoms of autism and other neurological child-development problems…" is from "Is Autism a G-Alpha Protein Defect Reversible with Natural Vitamin A?", by Mary N. Megson, M.D., and is available at http://www.whale.to/vaccines/autism35.html.

"My research shows that goat's milk will digest in a baby's stomach in twenty minutes, whereas pasteurized cow's milk takes eight hours…" is from *Journal of Dairy Science* 83 by Attaie, et al., (2000): 940–944; and Jensen, *Goat Milk Magic: One of Life's Greatest Healing Foods* (Escondido, CA:, n.p., 1994).

"Goat's milk has more buffering capacity than over-the-counter antacids…" is from *Journal of Dairy Science* 74 by Park, (1991): 3326–3333; and J. A. Gamble, et al., "Composition and Properties of Goat's Milk as Compared with Cow's Milk," Technical Bulletin No. 671, United States Department of Agriculture, 209280 (1939): 40–41.

"Goat's milk helps to increase the pH of the blood stream because it's the
dairy product highest in the amino acid L-glutamine…" is from "Studies
on Camel and Goat Milk Proteins: Nitrogen Distribution and Amino Acid
Composition," *Nutrition Reports International* 39 by M. A. Mehaia, (1989):
351–357.

"Goat's milk contains twice the healthful medium-chain fatty acids…" is from
"Goat Management: Lipids and Proteins in Milk, Particularly Goat Milk,"
by G. F. W. Haenlein, Delaware Cooperative Extension, and is available
at http://bluehen.ags.udel.edu/deces/goatmgt/gm-08.htm; and "Quality
Standards for Goat Milk," *Dairy, Food and Environmental Sanitation* 11 by
L. S. Hinckley (1991): 511–512.

"Goat's milk is a rich source of the trace mineral selenium…" is from *Journal of
Infectious Diseases* by Baum, et al., (2000); and *Alternative Medicine Review,*
Patrick, et al., (1999).

"Whole-milk butter produced from cows eating rapidly growing green grasses
is loaded with vitamins A, D, and E…" is from "Nasty, Brutish, and Short?"
by Weston A. Price, Weston A. Price Foundation, http://www.westonaprice
.org/traditional_diets/nasty_brutish_short.html.

Chapter 9: You Are What You Think

"Psychologist and author Dr. Kevin Leman said the best definition for stress…"
comes from *Keeping Your Family Together When the World Is Falling Apart*
by Dr. Kevin Leman (New York: Delacorte Press, Bantam Doubleday Dell
Publishing Group, Inc., 1992), 273, citing David Elkind, *The Hurried Child,*
rev. ed. (Reading, MA: Addison-Wesley, 1988), 42.

"It reminds me of buying the best DieHard battery you can find…" Ibid, 274.

"According to Dr. Michael D. Jacobson, author of *The Word on Health*, cortisol
and DHEA are two of the most critical stress hormones…" is from *The Word
on Health*, by Dr. Michael D. Jacobson (Chicago: Moody), 2000, 166.

"In contrast, studies have shown that people 'who experienced an episode of
deep appreciation or love for five minutes saw their IgA levels'…" is from
Ibid., 190, citing Research Update, Institute of HeartMath (Boulder Creek,
CO: Institute of HeartMath, 1995).

"A 2014 study of over 17,000 found that long-term exposure…" comes from
"Fear of Terrorism Increases Resting Heart Rate, Risk of Death," by *Science
Daily*, December 22, 2014, and available at http://www.sciencedaily.com/
releases/2014/12/141222165443.htm.

"Female death rates increased 77 percent, while male mortality increased
41 percent…" is from "Triggering of Acute Coronary Syndromes," *J Clin
Cardiol* 3 by J. Muller-Nordhorn and S. N. Willich, (2000): 73, citing J.

Leor, et al., "Sudden Cardiac Deaths Triggered by an Earthquake," *N Engl J Med* 334 (1996): 413–419; "Effect of Iraqi Missile War on Incidence of Acute Myocardial Infarction and Sudden Death in Israeli Civilians," by S. R. Meisel, et al., *Lancet* 338 (1991): 660–661; "Iraqi Missile Attacks on Israel: The Association of Mortality with a Life-Threatening Stressor," by J. D. Kark, et al., *Journal of the American Medical Association* 273 (19 April 1995): 1208–1210.

"Closer to home, where we are presumably safer, some experts have estimated that stress accounts for as much as 75 percent of all visits to a physician…" is from *The Word on Health*, by Dr. Michael D. Jacobson (Chicago: Moody), 2000, 161, citing Rollin McCraty, "Stress and Emotional Health" (paper read at Steroid Hormones Clinical Correlates: Therapeutic and Nutritional Considerations, Chicago: February 25, 1996).

"Just over 800,000 people in the U.S. die each year from cardiovascular diseases. Stroke kills nearly 129,000 people, and about 116,000 people die of a heart attack each year…" is from *Heart Disease and Stroke Statistics—At-a-Glance*, compiled by the American Heart Association and available at http://www .heart.org/idc/groups/ahamah-public/@wcm/@sop/@smd/documents/ downloadable/ucm_470704.pdf.

"The number of deaths from cardiovascular disease alone is one of every three deaths in America and more lives than all forms of cancer combined…" is from "New Statistics Show One of Every Three U.S. Deaths Caused by Cardiovascular Disease" by the American Heart Association News, and is available at https://news.heart.org/new-statistics-show-one-of-every-three -u-s-deaths-caused-by-cardiovascular-disease.

"Anyone—whether he or she is a health-conscious individual or a health professional—who doubts the effect of the thought life on physical well-being…" is from *None of These Diseases* by S. I. McMillen, M.D. and David E. Stern, M.D., (Grand Rapids, MI: Fleming H. Revell, 2000), 175–177, and 196.

"When the Nazis discovered that he spoke German…" is from *What You Don't Know May Be Killing You!* by Don Colbert, M.D., (Lake Mary, FL: Siloam, 2000), 94–95; citing George Ritchey and Elizabeth Sherrill, *Return From Tomorrow* (Grand Rapids, MI: Baker Book House, 1979).

"What was his secret? He told Dr. Ritchey…" is from Ibid., 95.

"Dr. Colbert observed, 'He had learned the secret that negative thoughts lead to negative words'…" is from Ibid.

"Psychologist Dan Baker discovered virtually the same thing after dealing with the devastating death of his infant son, Ryan…" is from *What Happy People Know* by Dan Baker (Rodale Press, 2003).

"At the time I wrote the original *Maker's Diet*, two Danish researchers questioned the validity of the placebo phenomenon…" is from *WebMD Medical News Archive*, by Andrea Braslavsky and reviewed by Dr. Jacqueline Brooks, May 23, 2001.

"Doctors McMillen and Stern noted a Harvard Medical School Conference in which a study was reviewed documenting that weekly churchgoers… is from *None of These Diseases* by S. I. McMillen, M.D. and David E. Stern, M.D., (Grand Rapids, MI: Fleming H. Revell, 2000), 200.

"Dr. Don Colbert noted that research conducted by the Department of Behavioral Medicine at the UCLA Medical School… is from Colbert, *What You Don't Know May Be Killing You!*, by Don Colbert, M.D., (Siloam, 2013), 92.

Chapter 10: Stop, Drop, and Roll!

"Dr. Mark Virkler, author of *Eden's Health Plan—Go Natural*, cited a study comparing two identical farming soils…" is from *Eden's Health Plan—Go Natural!* by Mark and Patti Virkler, (Shippensburg, PA: Destiny Image Publishers, 1994), 64; citing Max Gerson, *A Cancer Therapy* (Bonita, CA: The Gerson Institute, 1990), 176–181.

"As someone has said, 'The donkeys taught the atheists a lesson in practical theology'…" is from *God's Key to Health and Happiness* by Elmer Josephson, (Old Tappan, NJ: Fleming H. Revell Company, 1976), 163.

"Dr. William L. Esser followed the progress of 156 patients at his West Palm Beach retreat center in Florida…" is from *Eden's Health Plan—Go Natural!* by Mark and Patti Virkler, (Shippensburg, PA: Destiny Image Publishers, 1994), 186, citing Lee Bueno, *Fast Your Way to Health* (Springdale, PA: Whitaker House, 1991), 94.

"The pores of the skin, the mouth, the lungs, the kidneys…" is from *God's Chosen Fast: A Spiritual and Practical Guide to Fasting* by Arthur Wallis, (Fort Washington, PA: Christian Literature Crusade, 1968), 103–104.

"Lower cholesterol rates have no connection with lower incidences of heart attack or heart disease…" is from *Nourishing Traditions: The Cookbook That Challenges Politically Correct Nutrition and the Diet Dictocrats,* by Sally Fallon with Mary G. Enig, Ph.D., second ed. (Washington, DC: New Trends Publishing, Inc., 1999) 13, citing *Nutr Rev 52* by J. B. Ubbink (November 1994): 383–393.

"A brisk two-mile walk (with long strides and vigorous arm movement) every day increases enzyme and metabolic activity… is from "The Power of Walking," by Paul Chek, C.H.E.K. Institute, and is available at http://www.chekinstitute.com/articles.cfm?select=38.

"Functional fitness expert Juan Carlos Santana says it best…" is from "The 4 Pillars of Human Movement: A Movement Approach to Exercise Design and Implementation," by Juan Carlos Santana, M.Ed., CSCS, and is available at http://www.canfitpro.com/html/documents/Santana -The4PillarsofHumanMovement.doc.

"According to James White, Ph.D., director of research and rehabilitation…" is from "Jumping for Health," Morton Walker, D.P.M., *Townsend Letter for Doctors* (n.d.).

"The researchers conducted the eight-year study hoping to prove the value of consistent aerobic exercise…" is from *Eden's Health Plan—Go Natural!*, by Mark and Patti Virkler, (Shippensburg, PA: Destiny Image Publishers, 1994),132, citing "Exercise: A Little Helps a Lot," *Consumer Reports on Health*, volume 6, number 8 (August 1994), 89.

Chapter 11: Biblical Medicine: Herbs, Essential Oils, Hydrotherapy, and Music Therapy

"According to Rex Russell, M.D., thousands of herbal ingredients have been identified by chemists for their health-promoting qualities…" is from *What the Bible Says About Healthy Living* by Rex Russell, M.D., Revell, 2006, 198, citing David Darom, Ph.D., *Beautiful Plants of the Bible* (Herzlfia, Israel: Palphot, Ltd., n.d.).

"According to James Balch, M.D., author of *Prescription for Natural Healing*, herbs have an important advantage over isolated drugs…" is from *Prescription for Nutritional Healing* by James R. Balch, M.D. and A. Phyllis Balch, C.N.C., (Garden City, NY: Avery Publishing, 1990), 46.

"Medicinal herbalist James A. Duke, Ph.D., former chief of the USDA Medicinal Plant Laboratory…" is from *Herbs of the Bible: 2000 Years of Plant Medicine* by James A. Duke, Ph.D., (Loveland, CO: Interweave Press, 1999), 8.

"Aloe vera can be used for teenage acne, or you can try heating an aloe vera leaf and applying it directly to abscesses…" is from *Herbs of the Bible: 2000 Years of Plant Medicine* by James A. Duke, Ph.D., (Loveland, CO: Interweave Press, 1999), 33–36.

"Black cumin seeds taste hot to the tongue and are sometimes mixed with peppercorns in Europe…" is from *Herbs of the Bible: 2000 Years of Plant Medicine* by James A. Duke, Ph.D., (Loveland, CO: Interweave Press, 1999), 47–49.

"According to Dr. Duke, research has revealed five compounds in mustard that support cellular structure…" is from *Herbs of the Bible: 2000 Years of Plant Medicine* by James A. Duke, Ph.D., (Loveland, CO: Interweave Press, 1999), 54–55.

"Dr. Duke reports that USDA researchers discovered that cinnamon reduces the amount of insulin necessary for glucose metabolism in type 2 diabetes..." is from *Herbs of the Bible: 2000 Years of Plant Medicine* by James A. Duke, Ph.D., (Loveland, CO: Interweave Press, 1999), 77–80.

"Coriander contains twenty natural chemicals possessing antibacterial properties..." is from *Herbs of the Bible: 2000 Years of Plant Medicine* by James A. Duke, Ph.D., (Loveland, CO: Interweave Press, 1999), 85–87.

"Dr. Duke notes, 'My research shows that the spice contains three pain-relieving compounds'..." is from *Herbs of the Bible: 2000 Years of Plant Medicine* by James A. Duke, Ph.D., (Loveland, CO: Interweave Press, 1999), 93–95.

"The green leaves of the dandelion are rich in vitamin C..." is from *Herbs of the Bible: 2000 Years of Plant Medicine* by James A. Duke, Ph.D., (Loveland, CO: Interweave Press, 1999), 97–99.

"Dill seed oil inhibits the growth of several bacteria that attach to the digestive tract..." is from *Herbs of the Bible: 2000 Years of Plant Medicine* by James A. Duke, Ph.D., (Loveland, CO: Interweave Press, 1999), 109–111.

"Dr. Duke reports that Egyptian mummies exhumed after three thousand years..." is from *Herbs of the Bible: 2000 Years of Plant Medicine* by James A. Duke, Ph.D., (Loveland, CO: Interweave Press, 1999), 144–146.

"Dr. Duke reports that fenugreek's bittersweet seeds contain five compounds..." is from *Herbs of the Bible: 2000 Years of Plant Medicine* by James A. Duke, Ph.D., (Loveland, CO: Interweave Press, 1999), 119–121.

"Frankincense was also one of the four exclusive components used to make holy incense..." is from *Herbs of the Bible: 2000 Years of Plant Medicine* by James A. Duke, Ph.D., (Loveland, CO: Interweave Press, 1999), 132.

"Hyssop stops bleeding (as an astringent) and effectively masks odors..." is from *Herbs of the Bible: 2000 Years of Plant Medicine* by James A. Duke, Ph.D., (Loveland, CO: Interweave Press, 1999), 152.

"Juniper yields two forms of cade oil prized for use in men's fragrances, antiseptic soaps, and as a smoked flavor in meats..." is from *Herbs of the Bible: 2000 Years of Plant Medicine* by James A. Duke, Ph.D., (Loveland, CO: Interweave Press, 1999), 154–155.

"Milk thistle, which can be grown in home gardens, has been shown to support blood sugar and insulin levels..." is from *Herbs of the Bible: 2000 Years of Plant Medicine* by James A. Duke, Ph.D., (Loveland, CO: Interweave Press, 1999), 163–165.

"Peppermint oil is antiallergenic and is used in aromatherapy to stimulate brain activity..." is from *Herbs of the Bible: 2000 Years of Plant Medicine* by James A. Duke, Ph.D., (Loveland, CO: Interweave Press, 1999), 149–151.

"These days, myrrh used in a mouthwash can stop infections, and the herb is an effective treatment for bronchial and vaginal infections…" is from *Herbs of the Bible: 2000 Years of Plant Medicine* by James A. Duke, Ph.D., (Loveland, CO: Interweave Press, 1999), 170–172.

"Myrrh contains a compound called furanosesquiterpenoid, which deactivates a protein in cancer cells that resists chemotherapy, according to researchers at Rutgers University…" is from "Discovery Finds Myrrh Kills Cancer," by the Gannet News Service, *The Des Moines Register*, December 17, 2001.

"Mentioned in the Book of Job, nettles may contain substances that alleviate arthritis symptoms…" is from *Herbs of the Bible: 2000 Years of Plant Medicine* by James A. Duke, Ph.D., (Loveland, CO: Interweave Press, 1999), 179.

"Saffron was used medically in tinctures for treating gastric and intestinal problems…" is from *Herbs of the Bible: 2000 Years of Plant Medicine* by James A. Duke, Ph.D., (Loveland, CO: Interweave Press, 1999), 203.

"Spikenard oil may support auricular flutter or abnormal heart rhythm…" is from *Herbs of the Bible: 2000 Years of Plant Medicine* by James A. Duke, Ph.D., (Loveland, CO: Interweave Press, 1999), 210–212.

"Turmeric's essential oil has been proven to exhibit anti-inflammatory and anti-arthritic qualities…" is from *Herbs of the Bible: 2000 Years of Plant Medicine* by James A. Duke, Ph.D., (Loveland, CO: Interweave Press, 1999), 218–220.

"The Bible mentions at least thirty-three species of essential oils and makes more than one thousand references…" is from *Healing Oils of the Bible* by David Stewart, Ph.D., (Marble Hill, MO: Center for Aromatherapy Research & Education, 2002), 96–113.

"For example, one ounce of clove oil has the antioxidant capacity of 450 pounds of carrots…" is from *Healing Oils of the Bible* by David Stewart, Ph.D., (Marble Hill, MO: Center for Aromatherapy Research & Education, 2002, 18.

"Known as an aromatic stimulant and tonic for the digestive system, today calamus is used to relax muscles…" is from *Healing Oils of the Bible* by David Stewart, Ph.D., (Marble Hill, MO: Center for Aromatherapy Research & Education, 2002, 287.

"Onycha may help control blood sugar levels and can be inhaled for sinusitis, bronchitis, colds…" is from *Healing Oils of the Bible* by David Stewart, Ph.D., (Marble Hill, MO: Center for Aromatherapy Research & Education, 2002, 297.

"Cypress also promotes the production of white blood cells…" is from *Healing Oils of the Bible* by David Stewart, Ph.D., (Marble Hill, MO: Center for Aromatherapy Research & Education, 2002, 291.

"Nothing else will be as creative as worship, because you are doing more than expressing faith in the sovereign God..." is from *Worship: The Pattern of Things in Heaven* by Joseph L. Garlington, (Shippensburg, PA: Destiny Image Publishers, 1997), 9.

About Jordan Rubin

Known as America's Biblical Health Coach, Jordan Rubin is a *New York Times* best-selling author of *The Maker's Diet*, a wellness entrepreneur, TV personality, motivational speaker, organic farmer and founder of Garden of Life, Beyond Organic, and Ancient Nutrition. Jordan has spent 25 years studying naturopathic medicine, nutrition, and regenerative agriculture. Jordan and his wife, Nicki, have six amazing children.

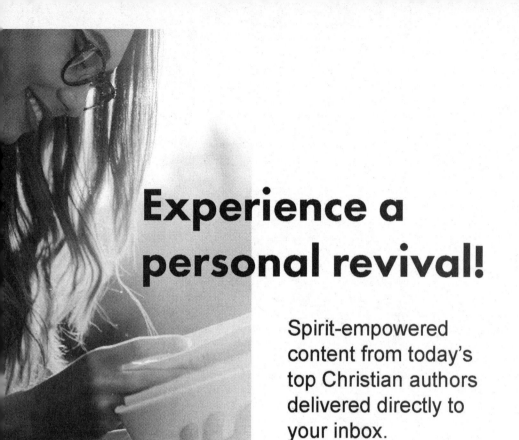
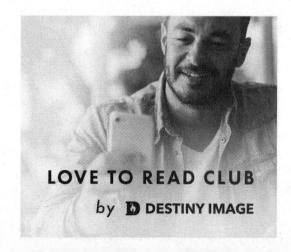